Counseling Persons With Communication
Disorders and Their Families

DEMCO

Counseling Persons With Communication Disorders and Their Families

FIFTH EDITION

David M. Luterman

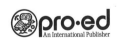

8700 Shoal Creek Boulevard
Austin, Texas 78757-6897
800/897-3202   Fax 800/397-7633
www.proedinc.com

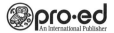

1984, 1991, 1996, 2001, 2008 by PRO-ED, Inc.
8700 Shoal Creek Boulevard
Austin, Texas 78757-6897
800/897-3202   Fax 800/397-7633
www.proedinc.com

Library of Congress Cataloging-in-Publication Data
Luterman, David.
    Counseling persons with communication disorders and their families / David M.
    Luterman. —5th ed.
        p. ;   cm.
    Includes bibliographical references and index.
    ISBN 978-1-4164-0369-2
        1. Communicative disorders—Patients—Counseling of. 2. Rehabilitation
    counseling.   I. Title.
    [DNLM: 1. Communication Disorders—therapy. 2. Counseling—methods.
    3. Family Therapy. WL 340.2 L973c 2008]
RC428.8.L87   2008
616.85'506—dc22

                                                            2007028916

Art Director: Jason Crosier
Designer: Vicki DePountis
This book is designed in Goudy.

Printed in the United States of America

3 4 5 6 7 8 9 10   17 16 15 14 13 12 11 10

To all clinicians who are willing to learn from their clients

CONTENTS

Foreword ix

Acknowledgments xiii

Introduction xv

1 Counseling by the Speech-Language Pathologist and Audiologist ◆ 1

2 Contemporary Theories of Counseling ◆ 11

3 The Erikson Life Cycle and Relationships ◆ 33

4 The Emotions of Communication Disorders ◆ 51

5 Counseling and the Diagnostic Process ◆ 77

6 Techniques of Counseling ◆ 93

7 The Group Process ◆ 123

8 Working With Families ◆ 145

9 Counseling and the Field of Communication Disorders ◆ 181

References 197

Index 205

About the Author 215

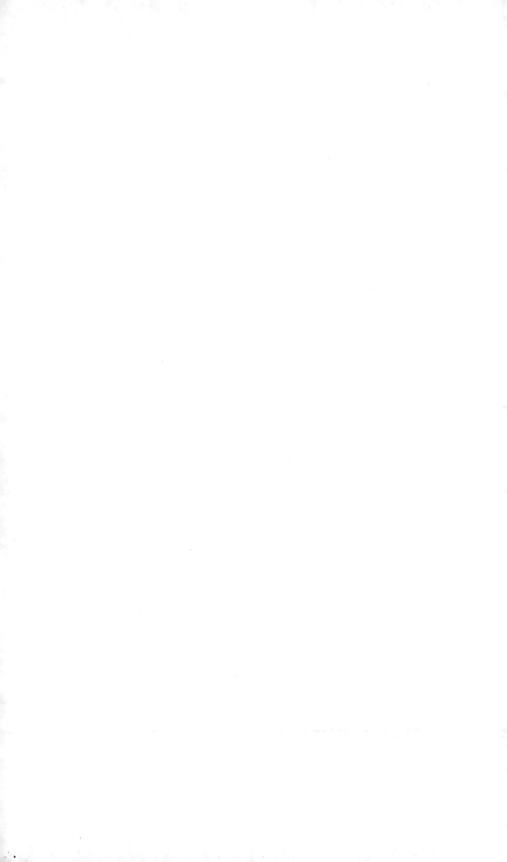

FOREWORD

The last decade has been witness to a revolution in the field of communication disorders. This revolution has been fueled by great advances in medical technology, computer applications, and "high-tech" instrumentation that have led to essential tools in research and treatment of individuals with speech, language, and hearing impairments. In this fifth edition of *Counseling Persons With Communication Disorders and Their Families*, Dr. David M. Luterman makes the case that there also has been another, more quiet, slower moving revolution under way, which is certainly not as headline grabbing and flashy as the technology revolution. The terms *raising of consciousness* and *gradual awakening* may more accurately reflect this increasing emphasis in communication disorders and other health-related fields. These terms refer to the awareness that treatment of persons and families with communication disorders should be, at its very core, a psychosocial process. David laments, however, that respect for the human service dimension of communication disorders has been slow in coming and continues to takes a back seat to a focus on technique and fact-oriented education and training of our students.

David was an early torchbearer of the humanistic and family-centered emphasis in communication disorders, and in this fifth edition, he once again persuasively argues that a clinician in communication disorders must be as skilled in working with and supporting people as in applying specific speech-language or audiological assessment or therapy techniques. Furthermore, David clearly communicates that for a clinician to be effective, simply having good intentions, or being able to empathize with persons and families challenged by a communication disorder, is not good enough. A clinician must have working knowledge of how a disability impacts a client and family, and how people generate their own capacities and strategies for coping (both adaptive and maladaptive) under what can be extremely stressful and challenging circumstances.

It is David's respect for the intricacy and complexity of the counseling process that makes his message so special. The prevailing attitude in many health-related professions is that supporting and counseling families is the easy part of the work and should not require special training. After all, we are in this profession because we care about people! Yet, to this day, I continue to be astonished by the "war stories" I hear from families about how the educational or health care system and its professionals (who probably consider themselves well-intentioned and sensitive clinicians) cause as much or greater stress for the family than the disability itself. Furthermore, when clinicians and students discuss the aspect of their work that is most challenging and therefore the source of most professional discomfort and anxiety, working with families and clients around emotional issues such as coping with a disability is invariably at the top of the list. Clearly we can do much better in working with clients and in training our students.

And this is the message that David infuses throughout this book. David's philosophy of counseling is, at its very core, deeply rooted in an optimistic belief in human capacity for growth and change. Consistent with his philosophy, this book does not focus on the "affected patient." The capacity for growth is an issue for systems of human relationships—that is, for professionals, clients, and their families, as well as for students in training. For persons and families affected by a disability, David believes that adaptation and coping is largely a process of making meaning out of difficult circumstances and, through this process, finding opportunities for individual and family growth. Because persons and families are so different by virtue of family structure, culture and religion, and specific circumstances surrounding the disability, by necessity, this process is highly subjective and individual. David contends that, with the support and guidance of a trained clinician (when needed), the ultimate outcome for a person or family may include empowerment in advocacy and decision making, a greater sense of confidence in coping with challenges, more fulfilling relationships within the family, and, in some cases, a reconsideration of one's life path. According to David, a belief in the basic competence of families must underlie the counseling process, for it is with this belief that families can be supported in making (and owning) the most important decisions regarding the affected person and other family members.

This same philosophy is the foundation of David's practices in training professionals in communication disorders and other health-related professions. That is, for effective counseling, the learning of techniques and facts is pointless without the development of a self-generated philosophy consonant with one's own belief system. Thus, David contends that students and professionals need to be able to make mistakes, learn from them, and not be afraid to feel the pain of their clients. The role of mentors and supervisors is to listen, support, and guide, but not to provide prescriptions and the "right" answers. It is through this process that students and professionals come to understand and accept their own personal and professional vulnerability, and ultimately to better understand those whom they serve. David argues that this process allows clinicians to discard professional masks and scripts in order to truly be able to support the individual and unique human needs of clients. I have observed that some clinicians may eventually reach this level of "expertise" through years of professional and personal experience. However, as David accurately points out, professional training and constraints inherent in work settings may actually impede such development and encourage a detached working demeanor. Fortunately, through David's writings, readers will benefit from the lessons learned from his long and distinguished career as a clinician and professor, as well as his own and his family's personal challenges.

For the professional and student, this book is, in part, about taking risks. The risks include reflecting deeply about how we relate to our clients and their families, and whether we take the more difficult path of understanding their pain and grief or remain objectively detached. The risks also include immersing ourselves in a world where simple prescriptions do not work and where there are no cut-and-dried answers. Yet, if we must avoid a "cookbook" approach, we must still be able to move forward and be effective in our relationships with clients and their families. The ultimate risk is to care too much about our life's work and the persons who receive our services. But with these risks comes the greatest reward—the sense that working with clients with communication disorders and their families is an integrated part of our lives, and part of our human growth and development, rather than simply a vocation that pays the bills.

For those students and professionals ready to take on these risks in the interest of their own professional and personal growth, I can think of no greater mentor than Dr. David M. Luterman. Largely due to the last 4 years of David's mentorship and friendship, I have grown tremendously in my understanding of, and therefore in my effectiveness in working with, clients and families, and with my students. Although I have worked closely with children and families for many years (under the assumption that I was a good clinician), I now experience a challenge and depth in my work that far exceeds what I knew in the past. Those of us who have been able to learn directly from David have been very fortunate. It is my sincerest wish that you who read this book also are ready to be nourished by the wisdom and experience that David offers, for I am confident that you, too, will experience greater fulfillment and challenge in your work.

In the Introduction to the second edition of this book, David stated that he would be content if his epitaph read, "He expanded our field by directing our attention to feelings and families." With this fifth edition, I can respond, "He continues to do so, and with great eloquence."

Barry M. Prizant, PhD, CCC-SLP

ACKNOWLEDGMENTS

With the extensive help of my son, Dan, I reluctantly entered the 21st century. Fortunately for both of us, my son has remained patient, and this edition was revised on my newly acquired computer, which I am coming to like when I can get it to behave. After the last edition, Dan was seeking a support group for the children of technologically challenged parents. Little did I realize that he can be replaced by his 16-year-old son, whom I am sure will be replaced by his 11-year-old cousin, who in turn will be replaced by his 3-year-old sister. This should keep Grandpa in business for a long time. I have hunted and pecked my way through this manuscript, desperately calling one of my children or grandchildren when I am in trouble. I owe them all a big debt of gratitude. Elizabeth Bezera, Emerson College librarian par excellence, was again an immense help in locating and supplying books and documents. My wife, Leonie, was a wonderfully compassionate critic and supporter.

INTRODUCTION

More than 40 years ago, I started my career as a clinical audiologist. At that time I thought I was interested in the precision and surety that working with machines seemed to give me. I soon realized that I was not a "machine person" but rather a "people person" and that the audiologic equipment was getting in the way of my relating to people. It was with some trepidation that I decided to come out from behind my audiometer and relate as a person rather than as a professional. The first outward manifestation of my slowly evolving inner changes was the willingness to wear nonwhite shirts; soon I went tieless. A few years later, I abandoned suits and sports jackets—the uniform of the male professional. A bit later I gave up all titles and prefer people to call me by my first name. These changes took more than 10 years to accomplish.

Rather than make a radical change in my life by moving to another position, I sought another way of relating to people with hearing impairment and their families. It became apparent to me that parents of children with hearing impairment were not being treated well. Everyone in the field of early childhood deafness acknowledges how important parents are to the habilitation of the child, yet parents are consistently kept peripheral to the educational process. I found that educational programs did what I did—namely, talked *at* parents and seldom *with* them—and no one was dealing with the parents' feelings. When feelings are high, people cannot retain content being presented, and all the information I was providing to parents went in one ear and out the other. So with a great deal of naiveté, I decided in 1965 to begin a parent-centered nursery program at Emerson College in Boston. In addition to a nursery and language therapy for the children, the Emerson program provided a once-a-week session designed as a parent support group, which I led. The program has continued to the present day and has afforded me a marvelous opportunity to grow both personally and professionally. Out of my experience came a book describing the program in detail, including procedures for counseling parents of children with hearing impairment (Luterman, 1979).

I found that people learned more as I allowed more affect (feelings) to enter into the relationships (e.g., letting parents cry), listened more, and dealt less with content. When the information was spaced over time, and when I allowed parents to work through their very normal feelings about having a deaf child, the parents could absorb and retain the information I and other parents were providing. I also discovered that people were not as fragile as I had thought (actually, it was my own fragility I had been worrying about) and that they could defend themselves quite well against my insensitivities and all-too-frequent lack of counseling skill. As long as I remained a caring, listening person, growth occurred within the relationship. I seemed to serve parents much better when I did not function in the traditional information-providing mode. As an added bonus, I found that my professional boredom was replaced by excitement.

The first edition of this book was initiated—as I suspect many texts are— when I agreed to teach a course on counseling persons with communication disorders and found that there was at that time no single, satisfactory text. For the speech pathologist it is becoming increasingly evident that more clinical time needs to be devoted to counseling. A recent survey of public school personnel indicated that as much as 20% of their time was spent in counseling (Flahive & Schmitt, 2004), yet the course work in preparing speech and hearing professionals still fails to reflect the importance of counseling. The ultimate purpose of this book is to demystify the counseling experience for the professional working within the field of communication disorders. It is my hope that, as a result of reading this book, clinicians will feel more comfortable in allowing the affect that is a normal concomitant of having a communication disorder to emerge in their clinical interactions. I hope this book will provide some insight into relationship building and its effect on the counseling process. By allowing more affect to occur in clinical relationships, speech-language pathologists and audiologists will find that their information-providing role will be enhanced and they will therefore be much more effective. I think they will also obtain more job satisfaction.

This text is not intended to supplant the clinical use of mental health professionals; they are trained professionals whose skills will be needed within a comprehensive speech-language and hearing program. I hope, however, that this text will lead to a modified use of professional counselors so that they can provide support and ongoing inservice training to speech pathologists and audiologists as they deal with the normal emotions surrounding a communication disorder.

One of my major justifications for writing subsequent editions has been to make the text more teacher friendly, in the hope that more instructors will be emboldened to adopt this text and offer a counseling course. (I have also written an accompanying Instructor's Manual, which is included on disk with this edition.) Alternatively, if programs don't offer a specific course, I hope they will infuse their communication disorders curriculum with counseling notions. To paraphrase Eleanor Roosevelt, in life it is easy to grumble about the darkness but much harder to light candles. To that end I used monies raised by the college to honor my retirement to fund a series of intensive workshops for college instructors on how to teach counseling. I hope to add more light to the field. Forty-two instructors have taken the course, and hopefully, as a consequence, more courses will now be offered. Those instructors who see the vital need for counseling education in our field seem to be a passionate minority but a growing one nonetheless and one that I hope will have increasing influence in the field. I am encouraged by a recent American Speech-Language-Hearing Association (2006) publication on the skills needed by audiologists providing clinical services to infants and children. Within the document there is an acknowledgment of the importance of affect counseling by the audiologist. Hopefully training programs will take action.

I have been teaching a counseling course at Emerson College for the past 25 years, and I have also taught intensive counseling courses at several universities. I am convinced that the most fruitful way to teach counseling is through a personal growth paradigm. The course itself needs to be a genuine encounter between the instructor and students to encourage students' personal growth. To be sure, there is a body of cognitive material that needs to be learned. At the least, our students need to be exposed to it; the content and the specifics of counseling technique, however, should not be the major focus of the course. Our goal as educators must be to give students a solid knowledge base that is integrated with and guided by their clinical intuitions and feelings. We must give our students permission to be authentic human beings in a genuine encounter with their clients. In Chapter 6, "Techniques of Counseling," the section called "Counseling Caveats" pulls together material that was scattered throughout previous editions of this text. I never like to stress the negative but I have found that counseling is as much a matter of what you do as what you do not do. The essence of counseling as I see it is listening deeply to clients and creating an environment of trust and then getting out of the way. It is a matter of students' shedding a great many preconceptions that are brought to the counseling relationship; it is my hope that this section will do just that.

In previous editions, Chapter 8, "Working With Families," was very much skewed to the families with young children with disabilities; it is now in better balance and shows how chronic illness of a significant adult can affect families. Shortly after my 65th birthday, my wife had a major exacerbation of her multiple sclerosis and became much more disabled, which necessitated increased caregiving on my part. The combination of diminished energy and increased caregiving led to my decision to retire from full-time teaching. I am now emeritus but continue to teach a counseling course and work with the parent group. Writing about chronic illness is not only a result of my personal experiences and professional practice as I continue to work with well family members, but a recognition on my part that chronic illness presents a huge challenge to our society which is not being met. It is becoming increasingly likely that every one of us will be either a caregiver or care recipient in our lifetime. Some will experience this early in life, as my wife and I did, and others will experience it later, but all of us will incur the increasing probability as we age that chronic illness will enter our lives. As a consequence, the work of professionals in communication disorders will increasingly involve contact with chronically ill persons and their families.

For me personally, since the last edition of this text, I have intensified my involvement with Buddhist philosophy. I find the notion of mindfulness and the gentleness of the approach immensely helpful in my personal and professional life. I find the combination of Buddhist and existential thought very helpful in promoting personal growth. I take every opportunity I can to expose students to these notions. Two books, Hanh's (1999) *The Heart of the Buddha's Teaching* and Kabat-Zinn's (2005) *Wherever You Go, There You Are*, have been very helpful in shaping my thought. I read portions of the latter book prior to meditating with my counseling class. I also have found the work of Cassell attractive. His book, *The Nature of Suffering and the Goals of Medicine* (1999), presents some interesting notions of the transcendence that often accompanies pain and suffering. This is something I have noticed in my personal and professional life. People often ask me how I have been able to work in this profession for so many years amidst so much pain and suffering. The answer is that I tell parents that I will share their pain as long as they will share with me their joy and growth. The latter are the moments of grace that make this profession worthwhile and have sustained me over the years.

At 72 years of age, I was beginning to think that it was time to rest on my laurels, but the dislocation in early childhood deafness caused by technological advances has stirred my passions again. Newborn screening has changed the diagnostic model from a parent-driven to an institution-driven one, with unforeseen consequences. Newborn screening is also conducted at a time that is not optimal for either parents or children. The cochlear implant in newborns has provided professionals, in many instances, a way to bypass or mitigate parents' initial grief reaction by holding it out as a cure; however, the technology often defers their grief to a later time when there is less emotional support for the parents. The implant itself has converted childhood deafness from an overt disorder to a subtle one that is not understood by many professionals and is not seen by parents until much later. Although I think the technology is marvelous and, when used appropriately, can mitigate the effects of early childhood deafness, it can sometimes have negative effects on counseling issues. Hence I pick up pen again, feeling like an old warrior tilting at windmills. I have devoted a section of Chapter 5, "Counseling and the Diagnostic Process," to dealing with technology and its impact on counseling. In that chapter I distinguish between the congenital diagnosis and the deferred one, each presenting unique counseling challenges. Newborn screening has converted early childhood deafness into a congenital counseling issue rather than a deferred one. I have also revised my thinking about the grief reaction in communication disorders and now see it as a chronic, episodic phenomenon rather than a stage issue. This discussion can be found in Chapter 4, "The Emotions of Communication Disorders."

The intervening years since the last edition of this book have been incredibly tumultuous for me. My wife of 44 years, Cari, died in March of 2001 from the complications of multiple sclerosis, which we had battled for over 30 years. The last 4 years were especially difficult for her and me, as she was almost totally disabled. The disease was unrelenting, and she did die at home as she had wished. Subsequently, in the fall of 2001, I met, at a Buddhist meditation group, and ultimately married Leonie, a wonderful woman with six children. With my four children and eight grandchildren, we tend to fill a tent. My life in my dotage is very full and incredibly happy. I never anticipated this outcome, having envisioned myself as an old man in a nursing home pushing a wheelchair. Instead I continue to write, lead parent groups, teach counseling, and give workshops. My attraction to Buddhism continues unabated both as a philosophy and as an ethical way to be on this planet. I see a huge application of Buddhism to counseling, and it is reflected in this book as in previous editions. I have recently taken workshops from Pema Chodren and Robert Thurman and have found their presence and writing most helpful. But above all, I have been gently guided on the Buddhist path by Leonie, who was recently ordained with the new name Samayadevi.

I have found that one of the gifts of being past 70 is that I have developed the wisdom of using my energy better even though it is diminished; I seem able to use it more productively than in my youth. One learns the art of pacing; things that seemed hard then are now easy. I just have to nap more. As I get older I also recognize fully how time limited I am and consequently I want to use my diminished energy and time well.

The nice thing about writing five editions of the same book is that you get a chance to refine and say what you want to say better. I have done just that throughout this text. It is a rare privilege and I am thankful to the publisher, PRO-ED, for giving me this chance. I do not anticipate producing any more editions, but given my previous experience, I never know. I guess the gods do laugh the most when we mortals make plans. We seldom know in life when there is actually a "last"; but this really does feel like a last to me. When my professional epitaph is written, I hope it reads, "He expanded the field to include feelings and families." This, however, may be a bit hard to get on the tombstone. This volume represents my 72 years of living and nearly 50 years of clinical work. It is my hope that you, the reader, can build on this.

COUNSELING BY THE SPEECH–
LANGUAGE PATHOLOGIST
AND AUDIOLOGIST

As an aspiring audiologist in training, I was taught that counseling was something one did after obtaining a careful case history and administering the diagnostic tests. Counseling was always information based and involved an explanation of the audiogram and recommendations for follow-through. I don't recall if we as graduate students were given an explicit injunction not to deal with the client's feelings, but we behaved as though we were. If a client displayed feelings (e.g., by crying), we were to refer the client to the clinical psychologist. The message I received in my training program was that client affect was the province of mental health professionals and that counseling by audiologists and speech-language pathologists was to be information based. This was essentially a medical model of counseling and indicated, I think, a desire to keep the field of communication disorders as a distinct entity as well as to avoid infringing on the mental health professions. It also, I think, reflected the lack of training in counseling in graduate programs at that time. Additionally, staying with content was professionally safe: With content, students could control the interactions; emotions were unpredictable and therefore potentially disruptive. With the medical model, students could adopt an attitude of detached concern and proceed to control the clinical interaction by delivering set speeches.

The medical model, at least among audiologists, remains the prevalent counseling approach. Flahive and White (1982), in a questionnaire study of 226 audiologists, found that a great proportion of their time was spent in informational counseling as opposed to personal adjustment counseling. The audiologists also reported that their training programs had exposed them to much more informational counseling (90%) than personal adjustment counseling (10%).

Many audiologists and speech-language pathologists receive no training in counseling. McCarthy, Culpepper, and Lucks (1986) surveyed training programs accredited by the American Speech-Language-Hearing Association. They found that only 40% of the programs offered a course in counseling within the department (36% had an out-of-department course and 23% had no offering at all). The most telling finding was that although the overwhelming majority of respondents felt that counseling was an important skill for speech-language pathologists to acquire, only 12% of the respondents felt that programs were effective in training students in counseling; a repeat of this survey (Culpepper, Mendel, & McCarthy, 1994) indicated little change in the number of counseling courses offered in training programs.

The lack of training is reflected in an increasing body of information indicating that audiologists are not effective in their counseling. Williams and Derbyshire (1982) questioned 25 parents of children with severe and profound hearing impairment under the age of 11 within 1 year of their having been seen by an audiologist. The results of the questionnaire study and personal interviews are startling and rather disheartening. The responses indicated that 84% of the parents were unable to understand all of the information they had been given, 72% did not know what a hearing loss would mean to their children, and 64% did not have a realistic appreciation of how hearing loss would affect their own lives. When asked by the investigators to restate the audiologist's explanations of the implications of hearing loss, 40% could not do so at all and 24% attempted explanations that the investigators felt were incorrect. Martin, Krueger, and Bernstein (1990) conducted a questionnaire survey of 35 adults with hearing impairment shortly after they had been given an audiological examination and had received content counseling from an audiologist. The authors concluded that "even when audiologists feel they have adequately covered all of the information during the audiological examination, the hearing-impaired adults' knowledge of this information is still lacking" (p. 32). Incredibly, not one respondent in their survey knew what an "audiogram" was after having just completed the examination. Haggard and Primus (1999) found that the standard methods of classifying a child's hearing loss may undermine parents' understanding and concluded that the standard way of classifying hearing loss evolved because of the needs of the clinician rather than the needs of the patient.

In an unpublished master's thesis, Lerner (1988) interviewed in depth the parents of a young deaf child (diagnosed at age 2 months) and the audiologists who had tested the child and counseled the parents. The parents were sophisticated, the father a physician and the mother a computer programmer. The audiologists were very experienced, both with doctoral degrees and 10 to 12 years of experience. The audiologists felt that they had done a good job of conveying the necessary information. The parents, on the other hand, were very dissatisfied, feeling that jargon was inappropriately used. For example, they felt the term "severe to profound" in describing their child's hearing loss was useless to them. (How often do audiologists use that terminology so casually?) What the parents most remembered was the tone of the comments, which to them was negative and pessimistic.

In my own clinical experience, this reaction is fairly typical of parents of newly diagnosed deaf children. When they leave the audiologists, they feel very confused and emotionally hurt and have not absorbed much of the informational counseling provided. When we are emotionally upset, we cannot process information very well; our brains go into a fight-or-flight mode, and we are ready for action but not prepared to process content. Parents invariably remember irrelevant details—the dress the audiologist was wearing or the color of a tie—and, although they retain little content, they always remember the emotional tone set by the audiologist—whether he or she was upbeat, hopeful, and emotionally supportive, or cold and factual.

Perhaps the crowning blow to our counseling egos was delivered by the study of Haas and Crowley (1982). The results of their survey indicated that parents of deaf children felt that the professional who provided them with the most meaningful information was the educator rather than the audiologist.

Certainly, some effective counseling is being provided within our field, and at times providing information is very appropriate. The audiologists in Lerner's (1988) study probably did have many successes. Nevertheless, we can be more effective in our profession if we are sensitive to the emotional state of our clients and feel comfortable in allowing affect to be a component of our clinical interactions.

It would seem that I am picking on the counseling skills of audiologists since all of the previously mentioned studies detailing the failure of counseling were related to hearing disorders. Unfortunately, there have been few studies of the effectiveness of counseling in speech pathology. These studies are badly needed. I suspect they would yield comparable results if the information provided by speech-language pathologists is offered without recourse or sensitivity to the emotional state of the client. A study done by Zeine and Larson (1999) on pre- and postoperative counseling for laryngectomees indicated that counseling was woefully inadequate: Incredibly, 21% of the laryngectomees reported that they were not aware that surgery would result in a loss of voice. This was a study that was a follow-up to one done in 1978. The more recent results indicated there was no improvement in the counseling provided over the previous study. The more recent survey of Flahive and Schmitt (2004) indicates that speech-language pathologists in public school settings are spending 20% of their client contact time in counseling, and that for every 7 minutes per contact hour spent in informational counseling, an additional 6 minutes were spent in personal adjustment counseling. This report would seem to indicate that speech-language pathologists are more willing to engage in personal adjustment counseling than audiologists. Clearly we need more recent research indicating what is actually happening in the field and how effective the counseling is.

In addition to counseling by informing, many professionals in our field counsel by persuading, which is a very seductive model of counseling. The underlying assumption of this approach is that "I as a professional have all of this information and experience. You as the client are ignorant of so many things that you need to know; therefore, I can make a better decision for you than you can for yourself." This approach often confirms clients' perceptions of their own limitations; they generally are feeling so inadequate and overwhelmed by the problem at hand that they often acquiesce to professionals' arguments and recommendations, basically letting the "doctor" decide. This is particularly true in the counseling of hearing parents of deaf children. A blatant example of counseling by persuasion can be found in the following excerpt from an article in which Dee (1981) describes her total communication program for parents of children with hearing impairment. (The article could just as well have presented an oral program. The issue here is the counseling style, not the methodology.)

> Most hearing parents of deaf infants need considerable help and guidance in developing clear and honest convictions about the real values of the total communication approach in the life of a deaf infant and his/her family. Even after their first pleasurable experience with total communication, during family sessions, when they have learned to use the simultaneous method to achieve a warm and loving communicative interaction with their infant, some of our parents will continue to undergo periods of doubt, uncertainty and even occasional resistance. Parents might also be struggling against non-supportive and/or antagonistic attitudes toward manual communication expressed by grandparents, relatives and friends. Furthermore, almost all parents cannot help but be vulnerable to the highly persuasive claims of the oralist. It is essential, therefore, to provide parents in total communication programs with a strong and convincing rationale for continuing to use this communication mode. A parent education program can provide yearlong opportunities for exploring and evaluating all that is "total" about total communication and for expanding and strengthening parental understanding of and belief in the emotional and educational gains that are the rewards of a total communication way of life. (Dee, 1981, p. 15)

This mode of counseling assumes that parents are weak and incapable of effective decision making: People generally conform to the expectations of them.

I, too, can recall persuading clients. A druggist with a very significant hearing loss once came in with his wife, who had been nagging him to get a hearing aid. Both the wife and I ganged up on him to persuade him to get an aid; she was arguing about how hard it was to live with him, and I was arguing about how difficult it must be at work and how hazardous it might be for his customers. He finally agreed to get the aid; a follow-up call 6 months later indicated that the hearing aid was in the drawer most of the time, and the wife was as frustrated and angry as ever.

In the 1970s, when audiologists were given the right to dispense hearing aids, the door was opened for the commercialization of counseling. Unfortunately, dispensing audiologists now have a vested interest that their clients obtain hearing aids. This makes counseling by persuasion even more attractive. In a book devoted to counseling and hearing aid fitting, Sweetow (1999) wrote that "counseling and selling cannot be separated. To sell we must present an image that instills confidence" (p. 9). This approach is the obverse of the counseling model I present in this book. Counseling, as I describe in this volume, requires that the counselor not have a point of view but rather that he or she employs selfless listening to enable the client to arrive at a decision that is self-enhancing. There is no "selling," and it might come to pass that clients decide not to purchase hearing aids. The mantra of the selfless counselor is, "This is not about me." This notion will be developed in more detail in this and subsequent chapters.

Counseling by persuasion is usually a poor approach because the clients never "own" their behavior. They do not take responsibility for having made the decision. The responsibility remains with the professional. My own experience has been that parents who have been persuaded to learn to sign with their deaf children are the ones who drop out of sign class early and seldom use total communication at home. Likewise, clients who are persuaded to get a hearing aid seldom wear it on a regular basis; they do not take ownership. True change comes from the inside when the person has made a decision and is willing to commit to it.

Another problem with counseling by persuasion is that it reinforces the client's feelings of inadequacy and becomes a confirmation of his or her own felt inability to make a good decision, and therefore the client's decision is to "trust the professional." This creates the dependent client—the one who is less apt to take any initiative or responsibility for solving the problem. The work is all left to the speech-language pathologist or audiologist who "knows better." This situation also tends to create fanatic clients—those who have been "brainwashed" and must now believe ardently in a particular approach, which has to be right because they have no other recourse, not having developed any confidence in their own decision-making skills. These are clients who do not think reflectively—they just believe. This is neither good education nor good counseling.

May (1989), a clinical psychologist, had this to say about advice giving:

> No deep understanding and very little empathy enters into the process. Advice (using the term in its everyday sense) is always superficial; it is a handing down from above, one way traffic. True counseling operates in a deeper sphere, and its conclusions are always the product of two personalities working together on the same level. (p. 117)

The two counseling approaches—informing and persuading—are not mutually exclusive. There are components of both in most medical model counseling sessions. After first informing the client of test results, the professional often sets about convincing the client of what to do about the data. A combination of informing and persuading counseling strategies can be very potent in the short term: When a professional overwhelms the client with information, the client's confidence is undermined, leaving him or her very vulnerable to being persuaded.

A third approach to counseling clients is one I prefer: counseling by listening and valuing. In this approach, the clients are seen as possessing the wisdom to ultimately make good decisions, and the professionals are seen as people who have the specialized knowledge to help illuminate the possibilities for clients. Counseling must always increase possibilities. The professional, by listening and valuing the client, bolsters the client's confidence so that the client ultimately makes good decisions that promote his or her welfare. For me, counseling is a mutually educative process that allows for the exchange of both information and affect. The aim of counseling is to help the client become better able to contend successfully with the specific communication problem at hand. Counseling as practiced by speech-language pathologists and audiologists should be problem centered with individuals who are emotionally upset by the problem at hand. This is opposed to psychotherapy, the province of specially trained professionals who are dealing with people who have chronic life adjustment problems. Many of the skills needed by both counselors and psychotherapists overlap considerably. It is the nature of the client and the nature of the problem that differ.

For us as speech and hearing professionals to be successful in counseling, we must help clients to become more *congruent*, or centered. A person's ability to function effectively in the world is a combination of the intellectual abilities (cognition) by which one processes data and the emotions (affect) by which one intuits the world. When one is congruent, one has equal access to intellect and to affect, and decision making becomes easier because of an increased awareness of who and what one is. One is able to respond to a situation with both intellect and emotion; the behavior then is always self-enhancing. Total congruence is an idealized state that for most of us is achieved only at very special peak moments in life. As professionals, we need to be always striving to become more congruent in our own lives, and we need to be always working to increase client congruence. For the purposes of this book, *counseling is seen as the process whereby clients are empowered to make informed decisions concerning their welfare; by doing this they assume ownership.*

Most people tend to have their own particular style of internal organization. Some people are high in intellect and short on affect, and others are inclined to approach the world and personal problems from a feeling orientation with little recourse to information. Invariably these opposites are attracted to each other as they seek to achieve congruence via relationship, if not in the world. This is important for professionals to note when counseling couples; invariably the two individuals in a couple will be approaching the situation from different perspectives. The stress of a crisis, which often occurs around a communication disorder, tends to push people further into their cognitive or affective orientation. The cognitively oriented individuals want "just the facts," and the affect-oriented ones are so full of emotion that they cannot deal with any facts. These differences present problems for the counselor.

For us to be effective at counseling, we must allow the affect-oriented person to ventilate feelings so that he or she can then begin to process the information that is needed, and we must help the intellectually oriented person gain access to feelings so as to become more congruent. This listening, valuing approach to counseling mandates that the speech and hearing professional be comfortable with the expression of clients' feelings and develop skills to elicit them. I have found that this approach to counseling is very often frightening to many in our field. If we are not informing and we are not persuading, who are we? Gregory (1983) described the problem well when he commented about counseling stutterers:

> It may be that giving information expresses dominance and giving direction is related to manipulation and control. Whereas we may view listening and attempting to understand as being indecisive and uncertain. For whatever reason many student clinicians and professional speech-language pathologists seem to find it easier to be a provider of information and direction. (p. 10)

The notion of allowing and eliciting feelings is also frightening to many speech and hearing professionals because of the mistaken idea that clients are emotionally fragile and that we can somehow hurt them by allowing them to talk about and display their feelings. The operative rule in counseling clients is that feelings just *are*. *Clients never have to be responsible for how they feel but always for how they behave*.

In a parent group I was just beginning to facilitate, a parent looked at me and said, "You are going to make me cry." I replied, "No. I am going to give you permission to cry," whereupon she began to cry. What I have to continually remember is that I am not putting the feelings in; I am creating the conditions where they can be expressed. Embracing one's painful feelings is the first step in healing.

If one thinks about it, how can we hurt people by listening to them and valuing them? E. Webster (1977) said it well when she wrote the following:

> If counseling means the imposition of prescriptions without care for the person for whom they are prescribed, one may indeed do damage. The non-accepting, non-compassionate clinician runs the risk of hurting parents, so does the one who focuses concern on the child to the exclusion of concern for the parents. The speech-language pathologist or audiologist who leaves to others the interpretation of the information his field has to offer may do parents great harm. The same can be said for the clinician with limited knowledge who gives faulty information.

> On the other hand, it is virtually impossible for one person to damage another by listening to him, by trying to understand what the world looks like to him, by permitting him to express what is in him, and by honestly giving him the information he needs. In this view of counseling, the clinician serves as an accepting listener. He delays his judgment and tries to accept parents as they are and as they will become. (p. 337)

I am encouraged by the recent skills document published by the American Speech-Language-Hearing Association (ASHA; 2006) for audiologists working with infants and young children birth to 5 years. This document finally acknowledges the need to access parents' emotions. This is the first official ASHA document that I could find that gives sanction to emotional counseling. I hope this can be extended to different age groups and different populations. The authors wrote the following:

> Content counseling is important for informational purposes, but emotional support and guidance through the grieving process also must be acknowledged and provided by audiologists. Furthermore, content counseling may not be successful with parents of newly identified hard of hearing children or deaf

children *until* parents have opportunities to work through their emotions. Audiologists must acknowledge parents' feelings, which can be intense, as they engage themselves in providing emotional support and guidance through the grieving process. (ASHA, 2006, p. 9)

This text is, I hope, designed to help the speech and hearing professional expand his or her scope of practice to include other possibilities for relating to clients beyond informing and persuading. With that in mind, we need first to examine theory and how that theory has implications for our field; then we can look at the applications of a listening and valuing orientation to counseling clients.

CONTEMPORARY THEORIES OF COUNSELING

There is an Indian parable about blind men and an elephant. Each man held on to a piece of the elephant and, when asked to describe the beast, each gave a very different version of the animal. The blind man who clutched the tail described the elephant as small, thin, and snakelike; the man clutching the leg described the elephant as very large and solid; and the one who held the trunk thought an elephant was flexible and strong. The point of the parable is that a person's view of reality depends on which part he or she is grasping and that perhaps every one of us has a limited view of reality at any given time.

A clinician trying to help a client manage change is much like one of the blind men in the parable. Clinicians operate from a theoretical framework that gives them a particular view of the "elephant." In practice, I think successful clinicians are eclectic in that they can and do mix their views, and are always evaluating which particular view is most useful in facilitating a therapeutic goal that fits the client context. Most counselors, however, still operate from a central tendency; that is, their theory of the therapeutic process serves as the organizing principles by which they tend to see client behavior.

With that in mind, let us examine the possible applications of four contemporary theories of counseling—behavioral, humanistic, existentialist, and cognitive models—to the field of communication disorders.

Behavioral Counseling

The behavioral model of counseling originated in the work of John Watson, with roots going back to Pavlov and his classically conditioned responses of a dog. Behaviorists concentrated on the strictly observable, with emphasis on external, environmental influences. (This emphasis was in sharp contrast to the subjectivity of the Freudian movement, which was beginning to invade American psychology around 1950, after many Freudians immigrated to the United States to avoid the Holocaust during World War II.) The leading proponent of behaviorism in the United States was B. F. Skinner. His seminal work, *Science and Human Behavior* (1953), became the basis of the clinical application of behaviorist notions to the alteration of maladaptive human behavior. Prior to the 1950s, behaviorism was pretty much confined to academic laboratory exploration using experimental animals (mainly mice and pigeons) (Rimm & Cunningham, 1985).

Skinner contended that human behavior is shaped by the environment that "operates" on it: If a particular behavior is rewarded—that is, reinforced by the environment—that behavior will be repeated. Reinforcement is either positive, as when a reward is given when the desired behavior is elicited, or negative, as when an aversive stimulus is removed as a consequence of the individual's behavior. (Negative reinforcement is not to be confused with punishment, in which an aversive stimulus such as an electric shock is applied as a consequence of behavior.) The reinforcement, whether positive or negative, must be applied according to a precise schedule. The timing must be exact so that the person associates the reinforcement with the behavior (this does not have to be conscious, as we shall see briefly), and the reinforcer must be either desirable to the individual or aversive enough to cause the behavior to change. Strict behavioral psychologists believe that there is no freedom or choice: All behavior, they believe, is a product of external reinforcements.

The behavioral therapist designs therapy based on the observable. This is basically an "engineering" model of facilitating change in that a goal is set and the task is broken down into a series of small steps. Each successive approximation is achieved by the judicious application of reinforcement. As long as the reinforcer is appropriate, the timing of its application is precise, and the desired behavior is within the physiological capabilities of the organism (e.g., one cannot get an elephant to fly, Dumbo notwithstanding), then the behavior will change.

The story is told, perhaps apocryphally, of a psychology professor who was lecturing his class on operant conditioning techniques. The class decided, on its own, to condition the professor. Every time he moved to the right, the class would sit up, take notes, and appear to be interested (powerful reinforcers to any professor). As soon as he moved to the left, they would slump in their seats and appear to be quite inattentive. It was not long before he was lecturing from the doorway situated at the far right of the room. When the class got bored with this, they modified his behavior by reinforcing any movement to the left, and pretty soon he was lecturing from the window. The professor, sophisticated as he was, responded much like any pigeon or mouse in a Skinner box, the apparent victim of the reinforcement schedule maintained by the class.

The fact that the behavior of humans can be changed as a result of the systematic application of reinforcement can be demonstrated both in laboratory conditions and in actual living conditions, and this approach has diverse applications to the field of speech pathology and audiology.

Application of Behaviorism to Communication Disorders

Behaviorism is a very attractive way of dealing with the deviant behaviors one encounters in a speech and hearing clinic. It provides a structured framework by which the therapist (especially the beginning therapist) can specify the particular behavior to be changed and, by breaking down the task into a series of successive approximations, can modify the deviant behavior. Progress at each stage can be measured. Perkins (1977) commented that

> because speech therapy is just as behavioral as behavior modification (the former derived pragmatically, the latter from operant learning principles), the same general therapeutic considerations underlie most of the methods for remediation speech. . . . In a word, the clinician must begin where his client can perform without failure and by careful selection of types and schedules of reinforcement, move step by step to the terminal goal. No step is taken until its success is assured. At the first sign of failure, the therapist mounts a strategic retreat to a point at which successful performance can be established. (p. 379)

Behavior modification techniques are used quite extensively in our field. The principles of behavior modification are relatively easy to teach to students, and the structure of the approach allays a great deal of therapeutic anxiety. The concrete nature of many of the techniques can be quite seductive to novice therapists. The 1970s, when behavior modification took hold in our field, seemed to be what could be called the "Fruit Loop" decade. One could rarely stick one's head into a therapy observation room without seeing a student clinician reinforcing a child's behavior with a Fruit Loop.

The literature is replete with behavior modification schemes. To name a few, Shames and Florance (1982) recommended a behavioral approach to shaping fluency in young stutterers; Moore (1982) recommended behavioral modification to eliminate or reduce vocal abuse; and Cottrel, Montague, Farb, and Throne (1980) used operant techniques for teaching vocabulary to children with developmental delays. Operant techniques have been used extensively in audiology to condition difficult-to-test populations to respond to sound (Lloyd, Spradlin, & Reid, 1968; Yarnell, 1983).

Among the many studies using the operant approach, two stand out. Stech, Curtiss, Troesch, and Binnie (1973) described the ways in which the client conditions and shapes the therapist's behavior. (The client strikes back!) Perhaps the ultimate study in behaviorism in our field is Starkweather's (1974) scheme to condition the student clinician, via earphones, while the student was conditioning the client. (One wonders who was conditioning the supervisor.)

Limitations of Behaviorism

The behavioral approach presupposes a very narrow view of the speech and hearing clinician's role and responsibilities, reducing the clinical task to one of dispensing Fruit Loops. The mystery and art of client–clinician relationships are not developed. This approach also leaves unattended the issue of carryover into the client's environment. Behaviorism would predict that a number of reinforcers in the client's environment are maintaining the deviant behavior, and these reinforcers are not addressed by working solely with the client. The behavioral approach is clearly able to modify superficial behavior but does not deal with such nebulous concepts as personal growth, self-esteem, and anxiety because it is hard to specify the overt behaviors; however, these concepts may have considerable effect on communication behavior and may be very useful for accomplishing therapeutic change.

A consequence of the unrealistic use of behaviorism to control behavior may be the loss of altruism. Philosophers and psychologists have postulated that humans are one species that demonstrates altruistic behavior—that is, doing good for the sake of doing good (although a strict behaviorist might say we do good because it feels good, and thus we get reinforced for altruistic behavior). Nevertheless, I think behaviorism would encourage a "What's in it for me?" attitude, which in turn would encourage superficial changes in behavior to conform to the extrinsic reinforcer. It remains to be seen whether a child, for example, can see good speech as something valuable in its own right or as a tedious prerequisite to getting a reward; if it is the latter, there is little likelihood of carryover outside of the therapy room.

It is also clear that humans do have choices about their behavior (a notion that behaviorists resist). If the college professor who was conditioned by the class had been made aware of what was happening, he could have resisted the conditioning and lectured from the center of the room, albeit discomforted by the fact that the class appeared to be asleep. It is this awareness of what is happening and the willingness to assume responsibility for behavior that will enable humans to control environmental reinforcers; however, the reinforcers may not be as powerful in shaping behavior in humans as they appear to be in laboratory animals.

Humanistic Counseling

Parallel with the development of behaviorism in the United States was the development of humanistic psychology, known as the "third force" in American psychology (i.e., third after Freudian psychoanalysis and Watsonian behaviorism). The theoretical and clinical underpinnings of the humanistic movement in the United States were provided by Abraham Maslow and Carl Rogers. Maslow (1962) postulated that humans have an innate drive to grow—he termed this drive *self-actualization*. The self-actualization drive is very frequently thwarted by teaching and parenting that direct the child to look to others for approval and wisdom. The goal of therapy is to help the person remove the barriers to the self-actualizing drive and learn to respond to the realm of inner promptings, where true wisdom lies.

A book written by psychiatrist Sheldon Kopp gives an excellent description of the humanistic therapeutic process. The book has the marvelous title *If You Meet the Buddha on the Road, Kill Him!* (1972), which comes from an old Buddhist admonition that any Buddha one meets on the road must be a false one, since the true Buddha is within oneself. As you can see, the roots of humanism are quite ancient. Lao-tze, a Chinese sage who wrote 2,500 years ago, articulated the humanistic credo so well when he wrote,

If I keep from meddling with people, they take care of themselves.

If I keep from commanding people, they behave themselves.

If I keep from preaching at people, they improve themselves.

If I keep from imposing on people, they become themselves.
(cited in Bynner, 1962, p. 32)

The application of humanistic principles to the clinical population is reflected in the monumental works of Carl Rogers. His seminal work, *Client-Centered Therapy* (1951), marked an ideological turning point in contemporary clinical psychology (Arbuckle, 1970). At that time, psychologists were concerned mainly with vocational counseling, intelligence testing, and personality evaluations. The client-centered counseling of Rogers, in contrast, placed little emphasis on diagnosis and testing—it stressed the quality of the interpersonal relationship as the means for promoting client growth. According to Rogers, there are three preconditions for change within a therapeutic environment. First, the counselor must develop an unconditional regard for the client so that the client feels free to express anything he or she wants to. This is fostered by nonjudgmental listening and valuing of the client within a relationship that promotes total acceptance. The client is never given a label such as "neurotic" or "mentally retarded" but is always accepted on his or her own terms.

Second, the counselor must practice empathetic listening—what Rogers referred to as hearing the "faint knocking." This is sometimes referred to as reflective listening and is the most seemingly teachable of humanistic counseling techniques. Unfortunately, if the technique is practiced without empathy, it will fail miserably, as it usually does in the hands of a novice practitioner who is focused on techniques and not on the client. (This is discussed further in Chapter 6.) In empathetic listening, the counselor reflects back to the client the feelings conveyed in the message.

The third condition, and probably the most difficult to achieve, is that of counselor congruence. Rogers (1980) wrote,

> when my experiencing of this moment is present in my awareness and when what is present in my awareness is present in my communication, then each of these three levels matches or is congruent. At such moments I am integrated or whole, I am completely in one piece. Most of the time, I, like everyone else, exhibit some degree of incongruence. I have learned, however, that realness, or genuineness, or congruence—whatever term you wish to give it—is a fundamental basis for the best of communication. (p. 15)

Counselor congruence demands that the counselor be in touch with his or her own needs and experiences. It suggests wholeness for the counselor to be "there" completely for the client. Armed, then, with an unconditional regard, empathy, and congruence, the counselor enters into a therapeutic alliance with the client so as to release the client's self-actualizing drive. Client-centered therapy assumes that, with these facilitative conditions, the client's resources for self-understanding and growth will be tapped and change will occur.

Application of Humanism to Communication Disorders

Speech–language pathology and audiology have a long humanistic history, going back to some of the field's earliest practitioners. Backus and Beasley (1951) felt that "speech therapy more and more is shifting away from an orientation based primarily upon devices, toward one based primarily on therapeutic relationships" (p. 2). Cooper (1966) reported that for stutterers, client progress was related to the nature of the affect interchange between the client and the clinician. He also noted that important similarities exist between stuttering therapy and psychotherapy. E. Webster (1966, 1977) consistently argued for a humanistic counseling model for the speech–language pathologist and audiologist, especially in relationship to parents, but also in therapeutic encounters. Caracciolo, Rigrodsky, and Morrison (1978) reported on the use of a Rogerian nondirective approach in the supervision of student clinicians. Their hope was that if the supervisor modeled the Rogerian approach to the student clinician, the would-be clinician could transfer this to the client relationship. In the field of communication disorders, probably no one has been as consistently humanistic in both clinical behavior and writing as Albert Murphy (1982), who wrote that

> happiness in the noblest sense comes in large measure through helping relationships with others, stretching our professional resources and the resource of the mind and the heart. Every now and then something in our deeper selves enables us to realize that what truly counts in life is not a matter of what is in you or what is in me but of what occurs between us. That divine spark of relationship may be the most fundamental life force of all. (p. 402)

Limitations of the Humanistic Model

The problem with the humanistic approach is how to apply it to the field of communication disorders. The concepts of congruence, empathy, and self-actualization are nebulous and are not readily amenable to measurement or, for that matter, to the teaching and training of student clinicians. Humanism requires a leap of faith: With the right therapeutic environment, the self-actualizing drive will bubble through. Thus, clinicians are left in a potentially uncomfortable, unstructured framework. Humanism demands that the clinician yield power to the client to determine the course of therapy—the "lesson plan" is thrown out or, better, is devised by both client and clinician in a spontaneous, egalitarian manner. Humanism places a great deal of responsibility on the client and demands a great deal of self-confidence on the part of the clinician.

Clinicians must learn behavior that appears to be contrary to what is usually thought of as professional. They must listen instead of prescribe. This approach demands that the clinician have an internal structure to allow for maximum external freedom. A humanistic approach is very difficult, especially for a young, insecure therapist who does not have the experience and confidence necessary to allow for an unstructured, spontaneous interchange with the client. It is also difficult to see how to apply the humanistic precepts to difficult clinical populations, such as very young children and adults with severe brain damage.

Counseling and Existentialism

Paralleling the development of humanism in the United States was the growth of existential philosophy in Europe. The existentialists emerged upon the rediscovery by the French intellectual movement of the work of the mid-19th century Danish philosopher Kierkegaard (Yalom, 1980). Existential philosophers were attempting to look at the problems of human existence without the comfort provided by traditional religious thought. They were very much a part of the scientific revolution that was taking place at that time and wanted to apply scientific thought to understanding life, which brought them in direct conflict with traditional religious thought. To the existentialists, the problems of living are related to the facts of existence—namely, that we must die, that we have freedom/responsibility, that we are alone, and that life is meaningless.

Existential notions also became the basis of an approach to psychotherapy. Therapists such as Viktor Frankl, Erich Fromm, and Rollo May began to use existential philosophy as a basis for understanding and examining the problems presented by their patients. Almost all of the existential therapists were latter-day psychoanalysts. In traditional psychoanalytic thought, anxiety is seen as the motivating force for a patient's deviant behavior. The source of the anxiety for the traditional Freudian is the conflict between the instinctual drives, such as Thanatos (death) and Eros (life), or between the id (the pleasure drive) and the superego (the social restrictions as incorporated within the infant by the parent in the form of the conscience). The resultant anxiety from these conflicts is the source of neurotic behavior.

Existential psychotherapy is a dynamic therapy that also postulates anxiety as the motivating force. For the existential psychotherapist, however, anxiety occurs when the individual confronts the facts of existence: death, freedom (which involves responsibility), loneliness, and meaninglessness. Neurotic behavior, according to existential psychologists, arises from the avoidance of dealing with the basic issues of existence. Existentialists do not take a developmental view of behavior in that they are not especially concerned with promoting insight into people's early history in order to understand current behavior. This is in contrast to traditional psychotherapy, which is historically based and seeks to help patients gain insight into their past in order to understand their present behavior.

Existentialism is a very "here and now" therapy that focuses on the present and sees the client's current behavior as reflecting some clash with one of the existential issues. The avoidance of the existential issues is viewed as creating the anxiety that ultimately gets individuals into interpersonal or intrapersonal difficulties. An excellent description of the application of existential thought to psychotherapy can be found in Yalom's (1989) book, *Love's Executioner*.

Existential Issues

Death

Death, the single most important issue of life, is a topic that most people avoid. Our death anxiety is best exemplified by that great existential philosopher Woody Allen, who commented that he just doesn't want to be there when it happens. Mitford (1963) pointed out how funeral directors increase their profits by catering to our death avoidance, basically by providing elegant clothing for the deceased, a soft and buoyant mattress, and of course the marvelous euphemism of a "slumber room" for the last viewing of the elegant coffin that contains the "sleeping" corpse. The existential philosophers tell us that if we continue with death avoidance, we will live a life with death anxiety—one in which we tend to postpone things and procrastinate without fully appreciating our everyday existence. If we do not recognize the boundaries of our existence, we tend to avoid enjoying the commonplace (after all, we are going to live forever!). The fear of death is greatest in those who feel that they have not lived their lives fully. According to Yalom (1989), "A good working formula is the more unlived the life or unrealized potential, the greater the death anxiety" (p. 6).

On the other hand, with death awareness, persons savor and enjoy every moment of the day. They are aware of how transitory and finite life is; they do not squander their time.

Yalom (1980) found the following changes in the lives of cancer patients as they came to grips with their impending death:

A rearrangement of life's priorities; a trivializing of the trivial.

A sense of liberation, being able to choose not to do those things that they do not wish to do.

An enhanced sense of living in the immediate present rather than postponing life until retirement or some other part of the future.

A vivid appreciation of the elemental facts of life, the changing seasons, the wind, falling leaves, the last Christmas.

Deeper communication with loved ones than before the crisis.

Fewer interpersonal fears, less concerns about rejection, greater willingness to take risks than before the crisis. (p. 64)

We are all terminal. How nice it would be if we could all develop death aware-ness without having cancer. Unfortunately, for most people, living with death awareness comes about only as a result of a life crisis.

Freedom/Responsibility

The existentialists are unyielding on the issue of responsibility; it is the basis of their therapy. To an existential therapist or philosopher, each person is respon-sible for his or her life and for constituting his or her reality.

Existence is you doing you! This uncompromising position can leave a per-son feeling very uncomfortable because there is no one else to blame for failure. For an existentialist, an individual is making choices at all times, including the choice of how to respond to an event in life. For example, although a person does not choose to be born deaf or to have a stroke, the person does have a choice about how to deal with it. David Wright (1969), a poet and a deafened adult, has written elegantly about his deafness and about disabilities in general. He found many positives:

> The handicapped are less at the mercy of vague unhappiness that afflicts so many, especially those without aim in life, whose consequent boredom pro-motes what used to be called spleen. The disabled have been given a built-in, ready-packed objective, which is always present; a definite impediment to get the better of. Like the prospect of hanging, it concentrates the faculties won-derfully. (p. 111)

As a counselor, one never feels sorry for a client, because the client always has a choice about what to do about the disorder; the responsibility of choice also provides an opportunity to grow. I think responsibility assumption is the basis of all change and growth. The first step in all therapeutic changes is responsibility assumption. If a person takes no ownership for his or her predicament, then how can the person change it? The hardest thing for clients to learn is that, from an existential point of view, there are no right answers in life; there are choices, and each choice has a consequence. Existentialists demand that we suffer the consequences of our choices. No wonder this is such an uncomfortable philosophy.

The pathology of responsibility evasion can range from the profound to the commonplace, and in some way, we all try more or less to evade responsibility. Erich Fromm (1941), in his classic book *Escape from Freedom*, asserted that, on a societal level, freedom engenders anxiety; hence, totalitarian forms of government developed as a protection against the responsibility required to maintain a democracy.

There is probably no more common occurrence of responsibility evasion than in the addicted personality of the smoker or the alcoholic. Smoking or drinking is not something that happens to a person; it is something a person does to him- or herself. The smoker or the alcoholic may feel as if he or she *has to* smoke a cigarette or have a drink, but the existential truth of the matter is that the person is choosing to smoke or drink. (There is evidence that alcoholics, in particular, have a different physiological response to alcohol than nonalcoholics, but this must never be an excuse; it still comes down to choice.) Addicts who are going to succeed in quitting are the ones who assume responsibility for their own behavior, recognizing that nobody is going to make the change for them. They also need a great deal of emotional support, such as that provided by groups like Alcoholics Anonymous. It is never easy to give up an addiction, but without responsibility assumption, it is impossible.

The existentialists are unyielding on responsibility assumption. One cannot even complain about the weather! I like the Ralph Waldo Emerson quote, "This would be a perfect day if we but knew what to do with it!" So, even with "bad" weather, it is our responsibility to make a good day of it. Another good quote is from Robert Louis Stevenson: "Life is often a matter of playing a poor hand well." Success comes from taking responsibility and thereby being self-reliant, as Holland (2006) found in her study of "successful aphasics."

Loneliness

Each of us is alone in the universe; after birth, we can no longer merge with anyone else. According to existentialists, almost all anxiety of childhood stems from the awareness of separation. The infant, who is not capable of surviving on his or her own, cannot bear to be separated from the parents because in actuality separation is death. Thus is born people's terror of separation and loneliness. Yet we are alone, and that crushing fact is central to existential thought.

Anxiety of loneliness gives rise to romantic love, the kind that is described in song lyrics, the kind that states, "I will die if you leave me." Romantic love fosters a mutually dependent relationship in which there is no growth. Scott Peck (1978), who devoted a considerable portion of his book *The Road Less Traveled* to a discussion of love, described romantic love as a biological "trap" planned by nature to ensure marriage, procreation, and thus the survival of the species. Romantic love may also be an evolutionary step on the way to mature love, which Peck defined as "the will to extend one's self for the purpose of nurturing one's own or another's spiritual growth" (p. 81). All definitions of mature love involve a separation that allows for growth.

The route to mature love may be through a crisis experience that brings us face to face with our existential loneliness. For example, Moustakes (1961), who has written extensively about the loneliness experience and how it relates to love, recounted his experience when he had to make a decision regarding major surgery for his critically ill daughter:

> It was a terrible responsibility, being required to make a life or death decision, for someone else. This awful feeling, this overwhelming sense of responsibility, I could not share with anyone. I felt utterly alone, entirely lost and frightened; my existence was absorbed in the crisis. No one fully understood my terror or how this terror gave impetus to deep feelings of loneliness and isolation, which had been dormant within me. There at the center of my being, loneliness aroused me to a self-awareness I had never known before. (p. 2)

Encountering our loneliness is a means of finding our unconditional regard for humanity. It is a "boundary experience," much like death awareness, which promotes self-growth. The love that stems from our loneliness encounter can be a love that comes from the richness of ourselves; in the giving, we renew ourselves.

Meaninglessness

For the existentialists, there is no extrinsic meaning to the world. For them, we are huddled on this planet hurtling through space in the face of cosmic indifference. The meaninglessness of the universe is central to existential thought in that the discovery of meaning for human beings is that which they construct for themselves. There is no "objective" truth, only a subjective one that is, therefore, highly individualistic. There is a world out there, but it is given form and substance only by human interpretation. In short, it is we who create God. (No wonder the existentialists got in trouble with organized religion.) In the face of a meaningless world, we must construct our own vision of the purpose and meaning in life, and we have choices about which view to take. Thus, one could take a traditional religious view (e.g., "We are here to fulfill God's design"), an altruistic view (e.g., "We are here to do good"), a dedicated view (e.g., "We are here to solve a particular problem"), a humanistic view (e.g., "We are here to self-actualize"), or a hedonistic view (e.g., "We are here to have a good time").

An existential therapist is always seeking to understand the client's particular view of the world. For existential therapists, there is never any judgment of good or bad; it is a matter of understanding what is and proceeding from there, and to always demand that the clients take responsibility for their choices.

Application of Existentialism to Communication Disorders

Existential thought has a very wide application to our field. The existential issues abound within all our clinical interactions. Since I have discovered the vocabulary and notions of the existentialists, I feel the excitement of Moliere's character, Monsieur Jourdain in *The Bourgeois Gentleman*, who discovers that he has been speaking prose all his life. Yalom (1980) commented that psychiatrists often do not deal with existential issues because they have not resolved them for themselves. I think that statement is partly true for me, but I have also needed the theoretical framework in order to see client behavior and to work through many of these issues for myself. Farran, Keane-Hagerty, Salloway, Kupferer, and Wilkin (1991) found existential issues abounding in the caregivers of patients with Alzheimer's disease. It was through suffering that the caregivers were able to assume responsibility for themselves and find meaning in their lives. My wife's illness also helped us to live authentically, making everything count, and gave meaning and focus to our lives.

The death issue is always present in our clinical work. In many cases, we are dealing with people who have undergone a traumatic change. All change involves a death in that we must give up and lose something. (We also get something, but we do not always recognize it at the time.) Parents of deaf children must give up the dream of having a normal child and also of their having a "normal" life. The client with aphasia and his or her family may have to give up the person as a viable communicating human being; this is a death. Many of our clients have literally had near-death experiences, especially those undergoing laryngectomies or strokes. This can leave them very frightened as they realize their vulnerability, or mobilized as they realize how little time they have left. M. Webster (1982), a speech-language pathologist who suffered a stroke, found that with recovery, "things like trees, flowers, sunsets and friends and loved ones are more appreciated" (p. 237).

Death awareness mobilizes the client and the clinician. When you are aware that death can touch you at any time, you abandon timidity; you want to extract the most from every encounter and you recognize that nothing is permanent. For the clinician, termination is an important clinical tool. All meetings need to have a very definite closure. Group meetings become more intense as the hour for termination draws near. Clients are motivated to work hard when they know that they have a very limited time to be with the clinician. There is experimental support for these notions. Shlien, Mosak, and Dreikors (1962) found that patients within a time-limited counseling program made more progress than did patients within a counseling program with no imposed time limits. Munro and Bach (1975) found that college students seeking counseling services showed significantly more gains in self-acceptance and increased independence when they were enrolled in time-limited therapy (eight sessions) than did a control group of students who had no time limitation.

When both clinician and client recognize that there is limited time, the emphasis in therapy becomes one of quality of endeavor. Time, per se, does not heal; only activity does. However, with an awareness of time limitation, there is an increase in activity and an increase in risk.

The freedom/responsibility issue is vital to any therapeutic progress and to any carryover of the behavior into the client's life. In my own observations of many therapeutic relationships, I have often seen clinicians fail to give responsibility for choice and behavior to the client. I often find that there is so much "rescuing" that the clients are not empowered and therefore do not grow. Geri Jewell ("Asha Interview," 1983), an actress with cerebral palsy, felt that the biggest impediment to her growing up was that teachers had low expectations of her and did not require her to assume responsibility. One sees the problem of low expectations repeatedly in the deaf population. White (1982) reported on a series of workshops he conducted with teachers and counselors at six schools for the deaf. Two hundred eighty-one participants were asked to rank 24 social competencies lacking among the deaf. The social issue ranked first by almost all participants was "taking responsibility for own actions."

Hornyak (1980), using the language of transactional analysis, pointed out the dangers for speech–language pathologists in "rescuing" clients, which robs them of their autonomy and keeps them feeling powerless. In the therapy contact, according to Hornyak, the client should be perceived as a human being who is not helpless.

When professionals become the ultimate rescuers of the people they are helping, they limit growth and keep clients from assuming responsibility for their own behavior. Somehow we must teach individuals who stutter to take responsibility for their nonfluency, clients with dysphonia for their vocal behavior, and persons with articulation disorders for their misarticulating. They must realize that the change comes from inside rather than from external sources. When clients recognize and experience their own powers and responsibilities, they can alter specific speech behaviors and maintain changes outside the therapeutic relationship.

The loneliness notion has wide application to our field. To have a communication disorder is to be cut off from contact with others. This is very anxiety provoking. It became apparent to me, as a practicing audiologist, that the underlying terror of progressive hearing loss experienced by some clients resulted from the feeling of being cut off and isolated. The major means by which we alleviate our interpersonal loneliness is verbal communication, and when that is difficult, we become upset. The child who would not let his mother out of sight because he could not hear her when she was in a different room in the house, the truck driver who burst into tears because he could not go to the bar with his cronies as he no longer heard the punch lines of the jokes they told, and the wife complaining about her hearing-impaired husband who refused to go out of the house because communication was so difficult for him, are, in one form or another, loneliness experiences. The stutterer who limits his contact with people, the laryngectomized adult who refuses to leave his home, and the individual with a cleft palate who avoids contact with people because of his discomfort with his speech and appearance are also very lonely.

Probably the loneliest of all is the adult with brain damage who is locked into his personal "cell" with blocked communication doors and windows. We must break through these doors, sometimes nonverbally with our touch. Alleviating a communication disorder is an incredibly tender and beautiful thing to do. There are not many more important gifts that we can bring to others. Any catastrophic change in a person's life becomes a loneliness experience because the person is cut off from all of the usual sources of support. Parents and friends seldom understand the person's pain of loss because they are so busy trying to make the person "feel better" that they do not respond to the grief; they also feel very awkward and do not know how to approach the individual who has experienced the tragedy.

Suzanne Massie, the mother of hemophiliac Bobby, wrote,

> The ostracism and isolation were almost harder to adapt to than the disease itself. More than ever we needed the help and comfort of close human contact.

> We needed friends. In our situation, they were essential. I cannot remember a
> single friend who was near us in the early days of Bobby's illness. . . . It was as
> though we were living on an island. (Massie & Massie, 1973, p. 148)

The encounter with crisis, as Moustakes (1961) found with his child, in itself, puts us in touch with our existential loneliness. How nice it would be to find a helping, empathetic friend at that time who just listens to us.

The existential issue of meaninglessness also emerges full blown from crises. Each of us has a cosmological view—that is, a way of explaining to ourselves how things operate in the world. Most people would like to impose on the universe an order and a rationality that existentialists tell us really does not exist. We need to find a reason for the tragedy, some way to explain it. The most common explanation is that God in heaven punishes the wicked and rewards the good: When something bad befalls us, we feel that we must have been wicked. (This is why in many cultures children with disabilities are hidden, because they are believed to represent some "sin" that the parent committed.) The converse view is that God is wicked, which poses a huge dilemma for most people undergoing a crisis in their lives; it involves a very painful reevaluation of their cosmological view. The deeply religious will often say, "This awful thing that has happened is part of God's grand design for me, but because I am only human I cannot perceive the total tapestry of God's intent."

Suzanne Massie, a deeply religious woman, had to wrestle with this big cosmic question of why:

> And yet the need to find meaning remains. . . . Why, God, why?

> I could not consider Bobby's hemophilia punishment. When I looked at my
> bright-eyed child, full of energy and drive, it was unthinkable that God would
> meaninglessly visit His wrath upon him. . . . Could it be to teach us suffering?
> The Russians saw in suffering a way to enlightenment. To them it was not a
> curse but a mystery with great potential for good. "Be glad Suzanne," Svetlana
> would say to me. "Be glad you feel deeply." "And remember," she would say,
> "You are a queen, because you are suffering." In the Soviet Union, a friend told
> me with respect, "Hemophilia is your family struggle; through it you have been
> able to glimpse the suffering of our Lord."

> In time I came to believe. In time I became grateful that we had been given the
> chance to see and feel so much. And I told Bobby this, that he had been given
> suffering earlier than many but that inevitably suffering and failure come to
> all in life. I told him he was fortunate to have had the chance to meet it when
> he was young, because those who meet it early are luckier than those whom it
> comes to later, when it often breaks them. (Massie & Massie, 1973, p. 148)

Vance (1988) encountered the love and the meaning that came with her recovery from a stroke. She wrote,

> But most important of all, I've learned how connected we all are to each other. . . . I've learned that my most important work is not what I write about, or what I research, but how I relate to others. I am connected to each person on this planet. My greatest work is to serve and love. I deeply believe we are all on a common journey. (p. 160)

All of our clients who are cognizant are constantly struggling with the issue of meaning. Those who are less religious are left with a void that they somehow must fill. Successful families and successful clients, as we shall see later, are those who find some meaning in the tragedies that have befallen them. Therapists must be willing to help the clients find their own meaning to resolve the "why me" crisis. This often means participating in or listening to "God talk," an area that is very uncomfortable for most therapists.

The existential issues also have cogency for us as professionals; through death awareness, we can restore our zest in our work. Clinicians who live with death awareness cannot be bored. Responsibility assumption leads to our personal and professional growth; through loneliness, we can find the mature love that truly nurtures our clients; and the resolution of meaninglessness gives rise to our commitment. I have found the field of speech pathology and audiology a rich opportunity for me to work through the existential issues. Working intimately with parents of newly diagnosed deaf children has added meaning and focus to my life.

Limitations of Existentialism

Existential therapy is much more a philosophy than a therapeutic technique, so there is very little for a clinician to grasp in working with clients; it demands that we stay with what we and the client know and can observe. Existentialists are very "now" oriented and are seeking to explain behavior in terms of the relevant existential issues, but there is no unifying strategy for evoking these issues. Clinicians are left to flounder on their own. Use of existentialism in clinical interactions would exceed the traditional boundaries for most speech–language pathologists and audiologists. For example, we would find ourselves involved in a great deal of "God talk" with many of our clients. Existentialism demands of us as individuals and as professionals a maturity that we may not now possess, but it will possibly be the avenue for our future growth. For me, an awareness of existentialism keeps me focused and grounded in what is important in life.

Cognitive Therapy

The cognitive approach to therapy offers a fourth view of the therapeutic "elephant." The underlying concept of cognitive therapy is that emotional disorder is basically a disorder of thinking. The cognitive therapist helps clients to identify the specific misconceptions and unrealistic expectations in their thinking that underlie their behavior, and then forces clients to test the validity of their assumptions against reality. It is a highly confrontational approach in that the client is always challenged to examine the underlying "irrational" assumptions that are reflected in his or her language and behavior. A cognitive therapist is not concerned with the person's past history, but is concerned only with the meaning that the client attributes to an event. A cognitive therapist is not directly interested in the emotions. The underlying assumption is that "as you think is how you feel," and if your thinking gets straightened out, so will your feelings.

Of the many cognitive therapists, the leading proponent was Albert Ellis (1977), the founder of rational-emotive therapy. He developed a list of the irrational ideas underlying the thinking of his clients, which in turn led to neurotic behavior. The following irrational ideas are adapted from his text:

- ✦ It is a dire necessity for an adult human to be loved or approved of by virtually every "significant other" in his or her community.

- ✦ A person should be thoroughly competent, adequate, and achieving in all possible respects if he or she is to consider him- or herself worthwhile, and he or she is utterly worthless if he or she is incompetent in any way.

- ✦ Certain people can be labeled bad, wicked, or villainous, and they deserve severe blame or punishment for their sins.

- ✦ It is awful or catastrophic when things are not the way an individual would very much like them to be.

- ✦ Human unhappiness is externally caused, and individuals have little or no ability to control their sorrows and disturbances.

- ✦ If something is or may be dangerous or fearsome, one should be terribly concerned about it and should keep dwelling on the possibility of its occurrence.

- ✦ It is easier to avoid certain life difficulties and self-responsibilities than it is to face them.

✦ An individual should be dependent on others and needs someone stronger than him- or herself on whom to rely.

✦ A person's past history is an all-important determinant of his or her present behavior, and because something once strongly affected his or her life, it should continue to do so.

✦ An individual should become quite upset over other people's problems and disturbances.

✦ There is invariably a correct, precise, and perfect solution to human problems, and it is catastrophic if this perfect solution is not found.

Applications of Cognitive Therapy to Communication Disorders

I think cognitive therapy is a model of counseling that is used a great deal in our field without our recognizing it as such. We use this approach when we set about to persuade clients, as when we list the reasons why someone should get a hearing aid or use an artificial larynx. We are not concerned with the client's feelings, assuming that once the person gets the appliance and sees how well it functions, his or her feelings will change.

A more systematic application of cognitive therapy has been with fluency disorders. Maxwell (1982) reported that a majority of his clients showed a significant reduction in the severity of their stuttering and a marked decline in speech-related stress under a therapeutic regime that employed various self-management and self-monitoring strategies. Emerick (1988) outlined in detail a cognitive approach to be used with adult stutterers.

I find Ellis's (1977) ideas immensely useful in almost all of my professional and personal contacts. Irrational ideas are reflected in the language people use to describe their problems. For example, clients often use "can't" when they really mean "choose not to," as in "I can't tell my pediatrician how angry I am" or "I can't use my new speech on the telephone." Translation: "I choose not to." The following are other language changes that I find valuable for clients:

✦ Change "should" and "ought" to "want to" or "do not want to," as in changing "I should use my new voice" to "I want to (or do not want to) use my new voice."

✦ Change "have to" to "want to" or "choose to," as in changing "I have to stay home and not meet people" to "I want to stay home" or "I choose to stay home."

◆ Change "we," "us," "society," and so on, to "I," as in changing "We are unhappy with this class" to "I am unhappy with this class (therefore I can do something about it if I choose to)."

◆ Modify "to be" verbs, as in rewording "I am a dumb person" to "I did a dumb thing and I am still a smart person."

◆ Change "but" (as in all the "yes . . . but" sentences) to "and," as in changing "I want to speak in public but I am afraid" to "I want to speak in public and I am afraid."

All of these linguistic changes force the person to assume responsibility for his or her behavior and for thinking clearly about that behavior. Underlying rational-emotive therapy, as with all other therapies, is responsibility assumption. I find that when I listen for the irrational assumptions that are reflected in the language of the client, and when I gently change the language, there is often immense benefit to the client.

I find that irrational ideas such as "I must be universally liked" and "A competent and worthwhile person makes no mistakes" are particularly valuable in working with student clinicians, as well as with professionals. These people generally try so hard to be liked that they are unwilling to offend their clients in any way. Thus, students and clinicians tend to meet clients' expectations rather than their own. The fear of making mistakes severely limits personal and professional growth and seems to be almost epidemic in student populations. I think that this is a direct reflection of the poor teaching methods that students have been subjected to—teaching that does not accept mistakes and incompetence as natural to the learning process. I always tell students, "It is only a mistake when you do it a second time." Almost every professional group with which I work is beset by these same issues, and professional growth is limited by the unwillingness to take risks.

Limitations of Cognitive Counseling

The rational-emotive therapies were developed for individuals whose emotions were in significant disparity with objective reality. The clients we are dealing with in communication disorders have very strong emotions, as I discuss in Chapter 4, and these feelings are based on a reality. It is very normal, very appropriate, and very rational to feel bad because you have a deaf child or an aphasic husband, or because you have had a laryngectomy. My own personal bias is that these feelings need expression and need to be acknowledged in order for counseling to move forward. A strictly cognitive approach cuts short the expression of feelings and moves clients quickly (I think too quickly) into the intellectual realm.

The other limitation of the cognitive therapies is the ever-present likelihood of getting into a persuasion model of counseling. A very fine line exists between cognitive restructuring and persuading. Counselors need to point out "irrationality" without prescribing. It is very difficult to do this. By prescribing, one may help to create the dependent client who does not think for him- or herself—the reverse of what any good counselor would want. The temptation to get the client to think as we do is very great, but this must be avoided if we are to be truly helpful. When we set out to persuade, we stop listening. We are so busy marshaling our arguments that we do not hear what the client is really saying, and this can be detrimental to effective counseling.

The Theories Compared

These, then, are the four views of the therapeutic "elephant" that I think have much relevance for our field. In theory, the approaches are very divergent; in practice, there are many more similarities than differences. To contrast them, I can use an example of a man going to a counselor to try to give up smoking. A behavioral therapist would devise a plan of cigarette reduction and periodic rewards for meeting the reduction criterion. A client-centered therapist would begin by asking the client what he thought needed to be done in order to give up smoking, and together they might devise a plan. The existential therapist would point out to the client that smoking is something he is choosing to do and perhaps he is now ready to choose something else. The cognitive therapist would direct the client to examine the irrational assumption he is making, namely, that lung cancer and all of the other known negative effects of smoking cannot happen to him.

In practice, latter-day behaviorists recognize fully the importance of the therapeutic relationship in promoting growth. Behavioral therapists have come to recognize that one of the first goals of the counselor is to establish a relationship with clients in which the clients feel free to express themselves to the counselors and in which the counselor is perceived as someone who is interested in attempting to help with the problem. It is also the clients who select the goals of therapy and, in concert with the therapist, work to change the environmental reinforcers that are maintaining the current self-defeating behaviors (Hansen, Stavis, & Warner, 1977). This view of counseling could be written by any humanist-oriented counselor. By the same token, Yalom (1975) (no behaviorist, he) commented that "every form of psychotherapy is a learning process relying in part on operant conditioning" (p. 57). Cognitive therapists and existentialists would agree wholeheartedly on the issue of meaning, and humanists are very much allied with existentialists, although they tend to be a bit more upbeat and less philosophically based than their existential counterparts. All therapists agree that no change can take place without responsibility assumption by the client. The particular routes to that goal vary, but many of the therapeutic roads cross one another.

No experimental evidence supports the superiority of any one of these counseling approaches. The variables that need to be controlled in order to determine scientifically which is a better approach (e.g., counselor competency, purity of counselor theory, level of client maladjustment, and degree and measurement of change) are currently so intangible as to preclude any meaningful research into therapeutic efficacy. Each counselor is reduced to selecting a particular approach because it is most congenial to his or her personality and worldview. The client behavior exists, and it is up to the counselor to choose a therapeutic lens through which to see it.

The general theory that a counselor holds about counseling is a reflection of his or her attitudes about humans and how they learn, change, and grow. Theory in this context becomes synonymous with "point of view," which in turn reflects how the counselor views client behavior. The problem with theory is that it can quickly become dogma and thus severely limit the response of the counselor. I think that each counselor must choose a particular way of approaching clients and then be willing to adapt within the context of the client–clinician relationship. My own personal view, which will be expounded later, is that all good counseling begins from careful listening, and when we do that, the client will teach us how to be most helpful.

THE ERIKSON LIFE CYCLE
AND RELATIONSHIPS

Among the pantheon of my personal gurus, Erik Erikson rates highly. The son of a Jewish mother, a Christian father, and a Jewish stepfather, he came of age in Germany during the rise of Hitler. As a youth he was an itinerant artist, a euphemism for a young man without much direction. He was employed as a tutor in a family that was friendly with Freud. Anna Freud, trained as an elementary school teacher, was interested in applying psychoanalytic therapy—developed by her father—to the raising of children, and became involved with the family that Erikson was tutoring. Erikson was swept up in the psychoanalytic movement and entered psychoanalysis—a requirement for anyone seeking to become a psychoanalyst—with Anna Freud. He finished his psychoanalytic training in 1933 and, because of the deteriorating conditions in Germany and his Jewish family connections, immigrated with his family to the United States. He worked in Boston for several years as a child analyst, one of the first analysts in the United States to specialize in children.

Erikson subsequently moved to the West Coast, studied the child-raising practices of the Sioux and Yurok tribes, and worked with the children enrolled at the Institute of Child Welfare in California. He became interested in how culture shapes personality and, with the eye of a painter and the training of a clinician, he observed the evolution of the life cycle from infancy to death. Among Erikson's many works, probably the most outstanding is his *Childhood and Society* (1950), in which he first delineated his observation of the life cycle. (Readers interested in further investigating the life and work of Erikson may want to read the excellent biography written by Robert Coles in 1970.)

Erikson's frequently used and quoted model of the life cycle is an immensely useful way to look at the developing ego qualities that emerge during eight critical periods of development from childhood to adulthood. Erikson felt that each successive stage has a special relationship to a basic element of society because the life cycle and humanity's institutions have evolved together. Each stage of ego development or "crisis" needs to be resolved, at least partially, before one can successfully move to the next stage. It is possible to think of the stages as a continuum in which the child establishes ego development features. This is a hierarchical structure in which each developmental issue is present in the previous stage and is further worked out in subsequent stages. A stage is presented as a duality, with the usual outcome as a balance between the two extremes. The reader needs to bear in mind that there are no distinct markers of stages and that the process of movement is not a straight line, as implied by the theoretical model. Cognitively, people like to have things clearly delineated; however, nature doesn't always work that way. The process of ego maturation is a sloppy, meandering one that becomes hard to describe and to grasp intellectually.

Erikson's Eight Stages

1. Trust Versus Mistrust

At this first stage, the infant must come to recognize that the world is basically a safe place—that needs are going to be met and that there is some consistency and order to the world. In order for the child to feel trust, the world must be predictable and the people who inhabit that world (mainly the primary caretaker) must be trustworthy and responsive in predictable and positive ways. It is believed that failure to develop this basic trust leads to the development of the severest forms of infantile schizophrenia.

2. Autonomy Versus Shame and Doubt

During the second stage, the child develops a sense of personal power, of having some control over the world. This begins as some motor control is established, and then as speech and language develop, the child can make wants known and begin to control others. Unfortunately, autonomy frequently emerges as a negative reaction to the desires of the parents; thus is born the "terrible two's." The child is working on establishing boundaries; meanwhile, the parents' task is to help the child develop a sense of autonomy with a benign conscience. If the child is controlled by shame, he or she will tend to become an adult who governs by the letter rather than the spirit of the law and suffers from compulsive behavior.

3. Initiative Versus Guilt

In the third stage, the child learns to be assertive, to take risks. The typical child moves into the larger adult society in an intrusive manner characterized by vigorous movements and occasional aggressiveness (especially toward siblings). There is also an insatiable curiosity manifested by the asking of endless questions. The parents' task is to allow the child movement into the adult world without clamping down so much as to limit initiative. Too many restrictions by the parents cause the child to develop a highly constricted conscience based on guilt, which limits the child's willingness to risk. Psychopathology at this stage leads to an adult who exhibits hysterical denial, who overconstricts him- or herself to the point of self-obliteration, or who develops a great many psychosomatic diseases.

4. Industry Versus Inferiority

The fourth stage coincides with the so-called latency period, generally when the child is between the ages of 5 and 11 years, although when one examines what occurs during this age span, it is clear that "latency" is a misnomer. Equipped with a sense of trust in the world and with some trust in self because of being allowed to develop autonomy and initiative, the child is now ready to learn formal skills. Society accommodates by providing the school, in its many manifestations, where the child learns the technological fundamentals of the society. The child acquires the tools that will be necessary in order to assume adulthood. The danger to the child at this stage is that a sense of adequacy may not develop, through either the failure of the family to prepare the child for school or the failure of the school to capitalize on the child's emerging abilities. An adult who has had difficulty at the industry level develops feelings of inadequacy compared with peers.

5. Identity Versus Role Confusion

Erikson's recognition of the adolescent experience as predominantly an issue of identity has received a great deal of attention and confirmation from developmental psychologists. The adolescent's task is to establish independence and freedom from the family and then, in the latter stages of adolescence, to establish a social role. The adolescent uses the parents as his or her first role model, and because the adolescent is also working on establishing independence from the family, will often appoint the same-sex parent as the enemy. There is a time when the parents are a total embarrassment to the adolescent. This is especially true for the oldest child; subsequent children have two models to work from (the parents and the older sibling), and these children are usually easier for the parents to deal with, as they fall somewhere between the extremes of the parents' and the oldest sibling's models.

Establishment of identity is a very complex process because it is also heavily influenced by significant adults outside of the family. Other family members, teachers, neighbors, and even characters in plays and movies all influence the adolescent's search for identity. Children raised in single-parent homes must use these outside sources to help them establish identity.

Identity is actually accomplished through life experiences. As we encounter situations in which we have some success and some failure, we get a more rounded picture of ourselves. Identity, then, is a constantly evolving attribute as we go through the life cycle. Failure to establish an identity during adolescence leads to gender confusion and role confusion.

6. Intimacy Versus Isolation

Erikson was one of the first child analysts to recognize that the life cycle did not cease at adolescence but continued into adulthood. Adulthood is not static, but rather is fraught with crises. As a child I often thought that when I was 30, I would "have it all together." I now recognize that growth is a continuous process: At times there are plateaus and at other times there are "breakup" periods; perhaps the times when we think we have it all together are merely interludes to be enjoyed and savored.

During the sixth stage, the young adult is an independent and self-governing individual; the task is to establish new ties to the world, free of the family relationships. These ties will evolve into the establishment of new primary relationships and of an occupation. Those adults who have a fragile sense of identity dare not enter into intimate relationships for fear of losing self, whereas those individuals who have little sense of self try to fuse with another and establish identity through the other person. In a truly intimate, loving relationship, both parties can and do maintain their separate identities. The young adult must find this balance—not an easy task.

Work also involves a fusion in which one must try to maintain a separate identity while feeling a part of the institution. An individual with a fragile ego becomes fearful of being swallowed by the institution and fails to commit, whereas an individual with little personal sense of identity tends to overcommit and merge personal identity with work identity. Neither solution is healthy; the failure to solve the intimacy crisis can lead to a deep sense of isolation and alienation.

7. Generativity Versus Stagnation

The seventh stage involves the need to ensure the existence of the species, either by literally becoming a parent or by sharing knowledge and skills with the young. It is the life cycle stage that is characterized by productivity and creativity. This is the stage of altruism wherein adults forgo their own personal needs to care for others. Generativity does not necessarily mean becoming a parent. One can figuratively instruct or care for future generations through work or charity. The mature human, according to Erikson, needs to instruct and teach. Thus is born the impulse to become a parent, write a book, compose a symphony, and so on.

The mere fact that one becomes a parent does not ensure that one has arrived at generativity. Some parents who have not resolved earlier issues around intimacy and identity are not able to give. They are still very self-absorbed and narcissistic, as one would expect at an earlier stage of ego development. In a similar vein, one's work can be long and strenuous but not very productive. Generativity enriches the individual as well as society; when such enrichment fails to take place, the individual stagnates.

8. Ego Integrity Versus Despair

For the aging or aged adult who has successfully negotiated the previous seven stages, this is the age of wisdom and detachment. It is the ability to see human problems in their entirety in the face of approaching death. One is able to love on a species-wide basis in the deepest sense. The mature elderly continue to grow and to adjust. The mature adult with ego integrity does not fear death and recognizes it as an integral part of the life cycle. Growing old does not guarantee that one will become wise. There are elderly adults who still fear death, who feel that life is now too short for them to engage in any new endeavor, and who are mired in despair. These are the elderly who have lived an unfulfilled life.

Life Cycle and Communication Disorders

Use of Erikson's life cycle model in the field of communication disorders has not been extensive. I have found one detailed application of it: Schlessinger and Meadow (1971), in their study of deafness and mental health, used the Erikson model as a theory for explaining the discrepancy between the normal potential and the relatively poor achievement of deaf people. Using their clinical experience, they found the developmental framework provided by the life cycle model valuable in looking at the deaf child. It appears that at each life cycle stage, the deaf child has a more formidable task in resolving that particular crisis than does the normally hearing child.

One might assume that the development of basic trust may be impaired in deaf children because of the delays and uncertainties in diagnosis of the deafness and the consequent anxiety of the parents. With newborn screening, the disruption in the bonding process and the establishment of trust can be compromised at a very early age. The parental grief reaction, which involves a great deal of anger and sorrow, may prevent the deaf child from receiving the consistency of parental care and responsiveness that is vital to the development of trust. When the deaf infant is undergoing diagnosis, the world must seem a very frightening place with many strangers and many unexplained parental absences.

The lack of clear communication can limit the development of autonomy and initiative in a deaf child. For example, parents cannot explain why a rule is imposed, and the child cannot ask the necessary questions to find out about the world. Parents also tend to limit their child physically because of the deafness, fearing that the child may not respond appropriately to danger. There is also high parental guilt, which is reflected in the attitude that "I let something bad happen to you once and I'm not about to let something bad happen to you again," and parents tend to overprotect.

At the competency level, the deaf child is again limited by poor communication skills and the overprotection of teachers and parents. Much of a person's skill acquisition is dependent on explanations. Teachers' preconceived notions of deaf children as low achievers may also limit the competency of the deaf child, who tends to internalize this judgment of the significant adults in the world.

Identity problems are particularly acute in the deaf child of hearing parents. In addition to the normal struggle to establish self, the deaf child has an apparent choice between the "hearing world" and the "deaf world." The child's problems are compounded if he or she has been raised orally, which too often involves a denial of deafness and the absence of a hearing-impaired peer group to relate to or any significant deaf adults to use as role models.

Schlessinger and Meadow (1971) observed that schools for the deaf have not equipped young deaf people properly for their introduction into the adult world. According to them, the young adult who is deaf is not prepared to understand the intangible rules of the hearing society and frequently regresses to a more dependent status, much to the chagrin of teachers and parents. It is also hard for these young adults to develop a sense of generativity because of society's discrimination against the deaf; love and work become very difficult under such conditions.

Almost nothing is known about the aged deaf; this is a largely unexplored area of investigation. One might assume that few deaf people achieve ego integrity, due to the increased difficulty that they experience at each life cycle level, or if they do achieve this level, they must travel a different route, one that is harder and more circuitous than that of the hearing population.

It would be very interesting to use the Erikson model on other populations with disabilities to see how they are affected; to my knowledge, this has not been done.

Life Cycle and Relationship Building

I have found Erikson's life cycle model to be a very useful way of looking at the development of a healthy counseling relationship, which is critical for growth. I find I can use this model at times to diagnose relationships that do not seem to be working—to find the point to which I need to return in order to develop a fruitful relationship. The life cycle notion helps me to understand how to build a relationship, as there seems to be a hierarchical function to relationship building similar to that in the life cycle model, in which each stage that is worked on has its origins in previous stages, and is worked out further in later stages. The following text describes how Erikson's stages can be used to build relationships.

Trust

Trust is the bedrock of a healthy relationship. Unfortunately, many professional relationships are not built on trust, and there can be no growth in relationships unless trust is present. There are three basic elements in building trust: caring, consistency, and credibility.

Caring is conveyed to the client in any number of ways, not the least of which is through active and sensitive listening. Kopp (1978), a psychotherapist, wrote,

> My first task was the creation of an atmosphere of trust within which we can enter into a therapeutic alliance. I begin by listening carefully to what a new patient has to say and to how it is said. I do not yet listen for the underlying dynamics that contribute to the patient's unhappiness. At the beginning, I am only trying to discover how it must feel to be that particular patient. For a while I do little more than try to formulate how the patient feels and to reflect those feelings back to the patient. It is enough that she finds that I am trying to understand how she experiences her life and that I help her to clarify her feelings without judging them. (Kopp, 1978, p. 81)

The key to the notion of trust building is nonjudgmental listening. If someone is willing to try to hear my fears and my concerns and responds to my feelings without telling me that I "shouldn't feel that way," then I can be more open and trusting. Joysa Post (1983), a speech–language pathologist who had a stroke and became aphasic, found that the quality she responded to the most in the clinicians who worked with her was caring. She needed a clinician "who cared and was interested in me as a person" (p. 23).

Trust develops when one believes that another person is reliable. Clinicians can earn trust by doing some very simple things. I start meetings on time and always end them when we have agreed to end them. If I cannot be at a meeting, I warn the clients ahead of time. If I have misrepresented issues or erred in some way, I apologize and correct the error. I try to be transparent about my feelings and my concerns. I also never tell clients anything that I cannot verify.

In the initial stages of a relationship, we as clinicians are granted credibility by virtue of title. People tend to give trust to someone who bears the title "doctor" (especially if a white coat is worn). Over time, however, credibility has to be earned. In part we earn it by what we know and how we convey it. The information given by the professional early in diagnosis is seldom retained by the clients because affect is so high. What is being worked on without either party being aware of it is the establishment of credibility. I will trust a professional if I think he or she knows the field even if at that point I do not have a sufficient corpus of stored information to evaluate the information being provided.

There are also all the intangibles of credibility establishment, which are conveyed to others by how I conduct myself, whether I seem to be in control of myself, and whether I share my information. Oddly enough, I have found that I do not lose credibility—in fact I gain it—when I am willing to tell clients that I do not know something. They are then willing to trust the other information that I provide. My willingness to tag something as unknown by me gives them the confidence to believe that what I do say is known. (Of course, there are times when what I think is "known" is not a fact; if I provide too much misinformation, I lose all credibility. It is my professional responsibility to keep my information up-to-date.)

One of the surest ways to lose credibility is by giving reassurance. Although the people we are dealing with frequently seek reassurance, when we give it, we also diminish ourselves. When we tell people "It will be okay" in order to help them feel better, they know that we cannot know that it will be better, and we lose credibility. I am always suspicious of anyone who seems to be telling me what I want to hear. At one level it is soothing; at another, though, I lose trust in what the person is telling me.

Autonomy

Autonomy in a relationship is the control that each party has; it is the feeling that I can make things happen that I perceive are in my best interest. Autonomy is always established in relationship to someone else; it is a bouncing-off that requires some form of negotiation with someone else, usually someone who is perceived as being more powerful. When the powerful other is the parent, then the child must be given some sense of control via some choices that are respected by the adult. This can save a great deal of grief. I remember walking one time with my wife and 4-year-old daughter at a fair, and it was quite clear we were all getting fatigued. I suggested to my daughter that she sit down, and since she was working on autonomy in a big way at that time, her only possible response was "No." My wife turned to her and said, "Alison, which chair are you going to sit on, the red one or the blue one?" and Alison promptly sat. She now had some control. She was permitted a choice, and her choice was respected. We all need that sense of control in our relationships.

Often, the powerful other in counseling relationships is the professional. How much autonomy do we allow in therapy? My observation of most therapy is that very little autonomy is granted to the client. I think this comes about as a result of the "lesson plan syndrome." Students in training are expected to enter therapy with specific plans and goals. This gives the therapist, especially the insecure beginning therapist, control of the situation. More experienced therapists will be flexible and modify a plan depending on the client. How many therapists, I wonder, develop the lesson plans in conjunction with the specific client, where both sit down and decide the agenda for that meeting? Client autonomy can be encouraged in little ways, such as by asking the client after a diagnostic evaluation, "What do you need to know?" rather than delivering a set speech and making all the decisions regarding the kind of information the client needs.

Professionals might have difficulty giving autonomy to the client for two reasons. The first involves time. When there is a waiting room full of patients, it is much more expedient to give the set speech and send the client out the door. This expeditious solution is usually the least efficient on a long-term basis, however, because the client will rarely retain the set speech and will generally return with the same lack of knowledge. What I do with clients is tell them, "I have 15 minutes [or whatever time I do have available]. How would you like to use this time?"

Second, the professional might worry that the client might not ask "the right question." In the context of a counseling relationship, there are no wrong questions. Generally, if clients do not ask the question, they are not ready to hear the answer, and the information provided is seldom digested. Gratuitous information usually serves to increase confusion and is rarely helpful. People will learn only what they are ready to learn and absorb. The best indication of readiness is the question. There are times when it is appropriate for us as professionals to provide information without being asked, and when this device is successful, it is generally because we have responded to the unasked question, which first requires sensitive listening.

Initiative

Initiative is an element of relationships that is closely related to autonomy. Initiative is the positive side of autonomy. Autonomy usually is established by the "no" in relationship to the powerful other and in some ways is easier than taking the initiative because the person does not have to take responsibility for his or her behavior. It is much easier to know what is not wanted than to take the responsibility for getting what is wanted. The professional fosters initiative by leaving spaces—essentially, teaching by creating vacuums. If I do not take total responsibility for what is going on, then the other person in the relationship has to act. It may seem damaging to my professional ego, but often the less I do, the more the other person learns in the relationship. This requires counselors to change some of the definitions of professional responsibility. Often the professional must "do" in order to satisfy the job description and the supervisors, while listening and responding are not always seen by either the therapist or the supervisor as being effective professional behavior. This attitude needs to be changed. Professionals need to learn to be comfortable with silences and with "not doing" so as to create spaces in which the client can take initiative. People grow through the acceptance of responsibility balanced by self-protection. Clients must learn to achieve this balance, and clinicians must help them in this task.

There are some dangers in this approach to fostering initiative. First, this behavior on the counselor's part violates the client's expectation of what a professional should do. (The client may ask, "Why am I paying you?") This violation will generate anger, which may or may not surface, that if not dealt with, can distort the relationship. The anger itself is a marvelous spur to taking initiative on the client's part, if the clinician can sensitively handle it. Second, by not acting, the counselor may lose credibility; there is a fine line that the professional must very delicately tread. The difference is in being responsible *to* (or responsive to) the clients rather than being responsible *for* them. Although I try to do 50% of the work and invite the other person to do his or her 50%, it is often hard to locate the therapeutic equator of responsibility.

Autonomy and initiative are attributes that are especially important for parents of children with disabilities to develop. They will need these traits when working with school professionals to devise educational plans for their children. It is very easy for parents to be intimidated by the confrontation with professionals. By now it should also be clear to the reader that initiative and autonomy are "loci of control" issues. Inner locus of control is obtained through the development of initiative and autonomy. (This issue will be discussed in more detail in Chapter 6.)

Industry

Industry is the relationship level at which most professionals seem to relate to their clients. There is clearly a task to be accomplished: a communication disorder to be overcome, a deaf child to be educated, a hearing aid to be obtained. Unfortunately, most professionals are so content or problem centered that they ignore the issues of trust, autonomy, and initiative. The professional's anxiety to alleviate the problem gets in the way of the establishment of the necessary precursors to effective joint work. The therapeutic alliance is not established when the professionals do much more than their 50%, and they often begin to complain about lack of client motivation.

Learning is obtained by any of three routes: by being told (lecture), by seeing (demonstration), and by doing. The most lasting way of learning is by doing. Unfortunately, for parent groups, in particular, professionals seem to use the lecture as the primary learning vehicle. Many parent discussion groups are really lectures provided by the professional on some topic that may or may not have been selected by the parent group. A lecture is a very inefficient way to teach because it assumes, incorrectly, that the audience is homogeneous in knowledge. The degree to which the learners have developed some trust will be reflected in their willingness to ask questions and take some initiative for their own learning. It is often difficult to get parents to ask questions after a lecture, when there is a low level of trust in the group.

As a teaching device, demonstration is very tricky. If it is not used sensitively, it can deskill the learner by increasing feelings of incompetence. I saw this occur in an itinerant therapy program when I worked with both the teachers and the parents of young deaf children. In this program, the teacher had to travel several hours to get to the parents' home and she had only a limited time to spend with the child. The teacher often brought in the child's favorite toy and invariably gave a successful lesson. The child was generally very eager to see the teacher, as she came only once a week and always had a new toy to play with, which she used skillfully. The lesson almost always went well, and the therapist would then tell the parent, who was observing, to continue working on this lesson during the week. When the parent tried to do the lesson by imitating what she had seen the therapist do, however, she usually failed. The failure occurred for a variety of reasons: The child was too familiar with the parent and resented the parent as teacher; the parent had many emotional issues about the child and often was not able to see the child clearly; and the parent was probably not very competent (why should she be?), which is why she was in the program in the first place. In itinerant programs of this sort, the parent is almost always programmed for failure, and thus begins to feel even more incompetent. My own bias about itinerant programs is that they should be entirely parent centered. I think that the teacher needs to see the parent as the recipient of the teaching and should rarely work directly with the child. To do this requires a large paradigmatic shift on the part of the teacher. She needs to see the parent as the client and view her own role as coach and collaborator with the parent. This is very hard for most teachers to see, as the focus of therapy for most therapists and parents is the child.

At meetings I always ask itinerant teachers if they are parent centered. Invariably they answer yes. I then ask them if they go into clients' homes with a bag of toys, and almost all do. I then ask, "If you are truly parent centered, then why bring in the toys? Why not go into the house and just work with what the mother has to work with and be her coach?" Some therapists respond with shock; others go and try working almost exclusively with the mother, reporting back to me how different the experience is and how effective it is.

A similar loss of competency can occur when a supervisor demonstrates to a student clinician a more effective way to establish the desired behavior in a client. This demonstration usually is done easily and effortlessly by the supervisor and leaves the student feeling totally incompetent. The supervisor may likewise feel incompetent when he or she goes to a conference and observes a master clinician at work. Demonstration, if not done sensitively, can have the opposite of the intended effect and leave the learner in worse shape. This is not to say that demonstration does not have a place in teaching—it can be a very valuable tool when there is enough trust in the relationship and when the learner already has established some self-esteem.

Doing is by far the most efficient way to learn, especially if one has a sensitive supervisor-teacher observing. Doing requires the highest degree of trust, for no one likes to appear incompetent, and the learner, by definition, is supposed to be incompetent. In order to learn, the student must be willing to reveal areas of ignorance to the teacher. Unfortunately, most educational programs reward competency and penalize ignorance; therefore, students learn to try to please the teacher by guessing what is in the teacher's head and by trying to appear competent when they are not.

Holt (1964) noticed that elementary school children, when given the task of trying to guess a number, would be disturbed by a "no" answer despite the fact that they gained as much information from a "no" answer as they did from a "yes." He concluded that one of the reasons children fail is because they are afraid of failure. No initiative can be taken unless there is a willingness to be wrong. For effective learning to take place, we must remove all penalty for failure and we must encourage mistakes (to put that another way, we must encourage learners to take risks). I have learned far more from my mistakes than I have from my successes. The failure tells me where my limit is and where I need to learn more. My successes, while gratifying, reflect skills that I have already mastered and no longer need to learn.

The unconditional regard and caring that I convey to the learners create the conditions that allow them to take risks. In short, there must be trust present for skills to be taught and learned. Each of these techniques—lecturing, demonstrating, and doing—has a value in learning, and each may be appropriate in a particular time and place. As we shall see in the next chapter, timing is critical.

Identity

Identity is very much role dependent; that is, how I define myself and how others define me will determine my behavior to a large degree. It is a function of the expectations that I and others have for that particular role. It is very easy to become role bound.

For example, the role of "parent" connotes someone who is not really involved in the educational or therapeutic process of the child. I remember once waiting outside my child's school to pick her up after an extracurricular activity. The principal, who did not know me, was concerned about a man lurking near the school. He asked me who I was, and I responded, "I am just a parent." Without skipping a beat, he responded, "What do you mean, '*just* a parent'?" We discussed that issue at length. Parents, as they usually define themselves in relationship to school, are an appendage of their child, someone who provides transportation, supplies, and lunch money, and who attends meetings to be told things about their child. They are always on the periphery of things and not really important to the learning process that is taking place in the school.

The role of "patient" also has a connotation of passivity, which is precisely why I have used the word *client* rather than *patient* throughout this text. The whole process of becoming a patient involves losing individuality. A patient goes to the doctor, receives a prescription, and follows it in order to get well. In a hospital setting, the patient is expected to be a passive part of the process while the professionals do the work. When patients refuse to cooperate—that is, do not conform to the role expectation—the doctors and nurses are immensely disturbed. Lear's (1980) book *Heartsounds* gives a remarkable view of the patient process from someone who has seen it from the physician's perspective. Her husband, a physician, found that when he became a heart patient, the attending physicians stopped listening to him and began treating him as a disease rather than as a person. His first act in recovering from his heart attack was to stop wearing the hospital johnny coat in order to retrieve some of his personhood.

The holistic health movement, which seems to be gaining more respect these days, puts the patients at the center of the healing process and requires them to take some responsibility for the course of therapy. I hope that this trend will continue in medical practice.

Probably the most role-bound individual in the therapeutic process is the professional. He or she usually is defined as the person who has the knowledge and the skill to make the other person "better"; therefore, the professional has the responsibility for making things happen, in short, for being "smart" and having the answers. Professionals are expected to write prescriptions and give advice. The manner of dress is usually narrowly prescribed (in some settings, it has to be a white coat), and the terms of address are carefully spelled out, usually with a formality that maintains a patient–therapist distance. Most of this self-protective behavior is taught at the training level and is readily adopted by the student clinician. A fully defined role is a means of gaining security: If one knows exactly what is expected, then one can conform to those expectations and behave appropriately. The price one pays for this security is rigidity in behavior that may very well limit growth. In fact, very often the traditional patient–therapist relationship has many features that limit the development of a healthy relationship; in particular, it fails in the responsibility-assumption area because the locus of control is external to the patient and in the hands of the therapist.

In the wholesome counseling relationship, where there are high levels of trust, where both parties are free to take initiative and have retained their autonomy, and where role definitions are not rigid, it might be very hard for the casual observer to decide who is the professional and who is the client.

Intimacy

Intimacy is very much tied to trust. When a high level of trust exists in a relationship, we can risk being open. Openness leads to a sense of caring and closeness. Intimacy also involves risk: The fear of intimacy often manifests itself in personally distancing behavior, which is often self-defeating.

In a counseling relationship, both parties need to feel that they can say what needs to be said. Only what is important between them is discussed and revealed. I do not have to disclose my bank balance in order to be intimate; however, when appropriate, I do need to relate—either verbally or nonverbally—how I feel about the other person. There is surety in knowing how the other person in a relationship is feeling. Intimacy also involves negative feelings. A great deal of trust is required before I can reveal that I am angry. Professionals who are role bound often feel that they do not have the right to be angry at clients. This attitude severely limits intimacy because no true intimacy is possible unless the full range of feelings that exist in a relationship can be expressed.

Intimacy carries with it the possibility of pain. As I become more caring and closer to people, I also leave myself vulnerable to loss when the relationship ends. Because of the anticipated pain of separation, many people limit their closeness. The price of this solution is an interpersonal loneliness. Here again, each individual must make a personal choice and resolve the interpersonal dilemma for him- or herself. Teaching—and, by extension, clinical work—is a very painful profession because many relationships are clearly limited in duration. The professional's temptation to limit intimacy and pain is therefore very great, which means that the counselor may avoid developing relationships that have maximum growth possibilities. I have found that when I limit risks, I also limit gains; hence, I have chosen to develop close relationships. The joy I have experienced during the semester is well worth the price I pay in June when both students and parents depart. Knowing that no relationships are permanent, I want to extract the most from each relationship that I have.

Generativity

Generativity becomes the outward manifestation of the skills learned during the industry phase. Now the client can go beyond the therapeutic relationship to demonstrate and develop increased skills in other relationships. This is the therapeutic carryover issue.

Out of the successful therapeutic relationship often arises the impulse toward altruism—toward making things better for others. It is no accident that many speech–language pathologists were themselves at one time recipients of therapy; although this might also reflect an identity issue, it very often is a reflection of the desire to give to others something of value that has been received. This is the noblest human drive.

I have watched parents go through the grieving process; they generally tend to progress from concern about themselves to concern about their child, and finally to concern about all deaf children. Parents are potentially a major resource for more far-reaching change, and their desire to help others can be channeled by the clinician to provide huge benefits to the community. Parents can and do become very active in promoting legislation and prodding bureaucrats to do the things that they should be doing. This very fruitful energy arises from a healthy therapeutic relationship that grows into the generativity or productivity stage.

Integrity

Integrity is the terminal phase of the relationship. Our job as therapists and teachers is to do ourselves out of our job, to no longer be needed. We are not doing our job well if we cannot let go of the clients we are serving, and, although this is painful, termination needs to be recognized as a necessary part of the therapeutic cycle.

Because of my own death avoidance issues, I once tried to keep termination discussion in my relationships to an absolute minimum. I came to see that this was a mistake. There is a need to "close up shop," take a detached view of the relationship, and process the experience. There is a need to bring the relationship to closure, to explain why I did or did not do certain things, to talk about previously concealed feelings, and to express often latent feelings of appreciation. I usually feel a sense of sadness at this time and a sense of loss. When I think about the new relationships that will be starting in the fall, I feel a momentary sense of despair at having to start the process over again. I wonder if the new relationships will be as satisfying. I also feel some excitement at the prospect of encountering new people and learning something more about myself.

Models as Clinical Tools

Models can be very dangerous if taken literally by the unwary reader, because they are a simplification of a very complex process. It might seem from reading this chapter that relationship building proceeds smoothly through the eight outlined stages, and that if a relationship is stuck, then all one has to do to diagnose the trouble is go back to the sticking point. In practice, this is not so simple: Relationship building is at best a sloppy process, with different stages being worked on at different times, not necessarily sequentially. At times, some issues are only partially worked out and then returned to; very often, several stages are being worked on simultaneously. Models become clinically valuable as conceptualizations; they enable us to talk about very complex phenomena by giving us a vocabulary. The reader must always bear in mind that the model is a simplification and not the event—it is but a particular abstraction of an event.

I have found the existential model and Erikson's life cycle model to be particularly helpful clinically. They complement one another nicely. The existential view focuses on current behavior that seems to be universal, whereas Erikson's model gives a developmental perspective within our culture. There are large areas of overlap between them. For example, Erikson's stages of autonomy and initiative are comparable to the existential issue of responsibility assumption; identity and productivity are intricately related to the meaning issue; trust and intimacy are very much part of the loneliness experience; and of course death is part and parcel of the ego integrity stage.

Despite the overlap, these models give us somewhat different views of human beings, and we can use whichever conceptualization seems most appropriate for describing a particular behavior. The reader must always bear in mind that there is no "right" view of human behavior—only a variety of ways to interpret a particular facet of behavior.

THE EMOTIONS OF
COMMUNICATION DISORDERS

Communication disorders are accompanied by strong feelings; this is true for both the client and the family of the client. Communication is so basic to humanness that when it is blocked or distorted, the people involved become emotionally upset. Often, clients' displays of feelings are very distressing to the speech and hearing professional, in part, I think, because of the lack of training in affect counseling. For most professionals in our field, there is an underlying supposition that the people we encounter are so emotionally fragile that any mistake on our part might send them over the edge. This makes us wary about exposing our own and our clients' feelings. As a beginning audiologist, I think I tried to forestall emotional displays because I was embarrassed by them and because I did not know how to react appropriately; I also felt vaguely guilty that I had somehow caused the pain, and in some ways I had, by being the bearer of bad news.

My difficulty in handling affect with my clients (as well as in my personal life) led me to employ all sorts of strategies to prevent feelings from emerging. I often used my sense of humor as a distraction designed to try to make people feel better. Alternatively, as a principal distraction, I provided information to keep people in their cognitive realm and away from feelings. I have learned, however, that the goal of counseling is not to make people feel better, but to separate feelings from nonproductive behavior. The feelings must always be acknowledged. I also have found that people have many diverse ways to make themselves feel better, and I can just allow that to happen. I learned over time that people were not really as fragile as I had assumed. The problem from the outset was my own fear and insecurity in exposing feelings.

It is always a mistake in any relationship to tell people, no matter how nicely we do it, that they shouldn't feel a particular way. When we do this, we help them to feel guilty about their feelings, as though they should not have them. Probably the least helpful thing to say to anybody is, "Don't worry about it," because then they start worrying about their worrying. What we really mean by "don't worry" or "don't feel that way" is that "your expression of feelings is distressing to me, so please stop." It is hard to see how this strategy can ever be helpful to people we want to help.

The operative rule for the counseling model described in this book is that feelings are neither good nor bad; they just are. They need to be acknowledged and accepted, but not judged. There is deep pain in having a communication disorder, and in most cases we as professionals cannot do or say anything that will take the pain away. The pain needs to be acknowledged for what it is, a very normal reaction to a terrible situation. Behavior, on the other hand, can be judged. We can see whether it is self-enhancing—that is, whether it is accomplishing the goals we would like it to accomplish. If it isn't, we can set about changing it.

This chapter describes the feelings associated with the catastrophic changes in families that are commonly seen by speech and hearing professionals. We examine the feelings and look at the behaviors that arise from these feelings. Behaviors confound the therapist–client relationship if the therapist does not understand the affective source of the behavior. I have found in my work with very diverse groups of people with communication disorders and their families that affect is universal, at least to our culture, and is not disorder specific. We as a species tend to respond in the same way to catastrophic events that entail loss and a change of identity. Although the display of the emotions is unique to each individual and the content is unique to each disorder, the grief process is the same.

Grief

In all change there is a loss. For anyone undergoing catastrophic change, it is the loss of the expected future that is grieved so deeply. For my first wife and me, it was the loss of how we envisioned ourselves after our children left home. Instead of having a very vigorous middle age, with many trips and lots of hiking and running, which we had expected, the reality was her disability; we never planned on her being in a wheelchair. There is always pain for the loss, and it is a pain that never leaves you. One father of an autistic child said, "When you first find out your child is deviant, it hurts like hell. Then it becomes a dull ache that never goes away." The pain of that loss never goes away. It is hard for most people in the helping professions to realize that it is not our role to take that pain away. Our role is to acknowledge the pain and thereby validate it.

The process of coming to grips with this type of loss is much like the response to a death because it is the death of a dream or an expectation. Much of the monumental work of Kubler-Ross (1969) in her astute observations of the terminally ill and dying is applicable to the losses experienced by persons with communication disorders and their families. However, I have found Kubler-Ross's stages of grief—denial, anger, bargaining, depression, and acceptance—a bit overused and too simplistic for a very complex process. I am always leery of any "stages" concept in the grief process. I think the process is basically amorphous, having fluid boundaries and being cyclical in nature, rather than being a straight-line progression. Tanner (1980) wrote a comprehensive article on the grief reaction and how this relates to the speech pathologist or audiologist. He commented that loss can be both real and symbolic, and that grief is not a single reaction but a complex progression involving many emotions and attempts to cope with loss. I find it clinically more profitable to examine the feelings in loss rather than seek the stages of mourning.

Friehe, Bloedow, and Hesse (2003), in a thoughtfully written article, describe grief in communication disorders as an episodic experience as opposed to a fixed-stage progression. I think they are quite right about this. In communication disorders we are dealing with a symbolic death, as in the loss of a dream of the expected future. This symbolic death creates chronic grief, as opposed to the real death experience, in which the body is put in the ground and then there are culturally sanctioned rituals to help the family assuage its grief. For the person with a communication disorder, there is no finality. The person and family need to live with it 24 hours a day, 7 days a week, and they are without the rituals to help ease the pain and manage the transition.

The episodic notion of the grief comes from the "trigger" events. What happened for my wife and me after the intense pain of the initial diagnosis was that we settled into a life of "disability normal." By this I mean that we just adjusted to her level of disability, and this became our day-to-day reality. This is like living in a bubble of denial; your head is down and you just go about living your life not thinking about how out of the mainstream you are. The pain is put on hold. It wasn't until there needed to be a change in our reality, such as when she moved from crutches to a wheelchair, that we were jolted and we realized again how abnormal our life was. Trigger events could be as simple as seeing a couple of a similar age as us on a street walking together. For parents of a deaf child living "deaf normal," a trigger event may be as simple as going to a birthday party and seeing how well the other children are talking, and then the disability hits them in the face again. The grief is chronic and episodic for the families struggling with communication disorders. It is what the father of an autistic child meant when he said, "The pain never goes away." The grief is short term; however, because there are always trigger events, mourning is lifelong.

Behaviorally, the bereaved can get stuck in their loss and not see any positives because they are so busy mourning what they have lost and fail to see what is still there. I sometimes use the following piece, by Emily Perle Kinsley, in parent groups to help facilitate the grief process—some parents like it, while others think it is awful. It is always a timing call. When parents are beginning to look beyond the disability, they like it; when still stuck in it, they hate it.

Welcome to Holland

When you're going to have a baby, it's like planning a wonderful vacation trip to Italy. You get a bunch of guide books and make all your plans. The Coliseum . . . The Michelangelo David . . . the gondolas in Venice. You get a book of handy phrases and learn how to say a few words in Italian. It's all very exciting.

Finally, the time comes for your trip. You pack your bags and off you go.

Several hours later, the plane lands. The stewardess comes in and says, "Welcome to Holland."

"Holland?!?" you say. "Holland?? I signed up for Italy! All my life I've dreamed of going to Italy!"

"I'm sorry," she says. "There's been a change and we've landed in Holland."

"But I don't know anything about Holland! I never thought of going to Holland. I have no idea what you do in Holland!"

What's important is that they haven't taken you to a terrible ugly place, full of famine, pestilence and disease. It's just—a *different* place.

So you have to go out and buy a whole new set of guide books . . . you have to learn a whole new language . . . and you'll meet a whole new bunch of people you would never have met otherwise.

Holland. It's slower-paced than Italy, less flashy than Italy . . . but after you've been there for a while, and you've had a chance to catch your breath, you look around and begin to discover that Holland has windmills . . . and Holland has tulips . . . Holland even has Rembrandts.

But everyone you know is busy coming and going from Italy . . . and they're all bragging about what a great time they had there. And for the rest of your life you will say, "Yes, that's where I was supposed to go. That's what I had planned." And the pain of that will never, ever, ever, ever go away. And you must accept that pain—because the loss of that dream is a very significant loss.

But . . . if you spend your time mourning the fact that you never got to go to Italy, you may never be available to enjoy the very *lovely*, very *special* things about Holland.

—*Emily Perle Kinsley*
(Copyright 1987 by the author. Reprinted with permission.)

So many mourners feel stuck in "Holland"—always bemoaning the fact that they are not in "Italy." The ultimate goal of counseling, as I see it, is to help people recognize what Holland has to offer, and although they may always regret the lost trip to Italy, they can learn to appreciate what they have in Holland.

Inadequacy

Anyone faced with a daunting change in life will experience feelings of being overwhelmed by and inadequate to deal with the new challenges posed by the catastrophic event. Parents of children with disabilities in particular feel overwhelmed. The responsibility is awesome. When parents are told that their child has a disability—a statement usually accompanied by an admonition of some helping professionals that "if this child is to succeed, then it is up to the parents"—the normal terror of parenthood is increased fourfold.

A direct concomitant of the feeling of being overwhelmed is the desire to be rescued. The rescue notion, on the parents' part, manifests itself in many ways. A frequent fantasy that emerges in parent support groups is, "Wouldn't it be nice if someone came and took my child and brought him back when he was 18, all civilized and talking beautifully!" This fantasy is usually presented with a laugh, but it does reflect the underlying insecurity and inadequacy felt by the parents. (This is also the appeal of the residential school, which will take the responsibility from the parents.)

In one parent group, a father beseeched me to be the quarterback of his team. When I declined, he offered me the position of coach, which I also declined. The only role in his personal odyssey that I was willing to accept was that of enthusiastic fan. I told him that I would be in the stands, rooting hard and sharing all my information, but that he would have to select and send in his own plays. When the professional calls the plays, the parents become the spectators and assume no responsibility for the outcome. They may either praise or blame the coach, but they are not involved. Spectators are passive and seldom grow or learn very much.

Unfortunately, too many professionals in our field are willing to call the plays (see, e.g., the Dee, 1981, article cited in Chapter 1). It is a very difficult trap to avoid. The people whom we are pledged to help are coming to us in a great deal of pain and are feeling inadequate and overwhelmed by the responsibility. They often say, "I'm *just* a parent; you're the professional." (The previous statement is known as a "hook." This is the way clients who are in a dependent relationship try to "hook" the professional into assuming responsibility. The hook must be avoided at all costs in order to encourage an empowered family.) Because counselors have a great deal of information and compassion, they may feel tempted to take the responsibility from the parents and rescue them. To do so, however, creates spectators of the parents (or anyone else facing a marked life change).

Probably the best example in contemporary literature of the ultimate rescuer is in the story of Annie Sullivan and Helen Keller. Annie Sullivan, especially as depicted in the film *The Miracle Worker*, became a role model and a vocational inspiration for many in our profession. A biography written by Lash (1980) gives a more complete story of the Annie Sullivan–Mrs. Keller–Helen Keller triangle. Annie Sullivan had a very deprived childhood. After her mother's death, the 6-year-old Annie and her 4-year-old brother were placed in a home for the indigent by their alcoholic father. Her brother died shortly after being placed in the facility, and Annie literally had nothing while growing up among destitute, elderly people. Because of a visual problem, she was sent to the Perkins School for the Blind in Boston and received her education among an institutionalized blind population. The plea for help from the Kellers arrived as Annie was graduating, and she was sent to Alabama to rescue the family. It is easy to imagine the young Annie Sullivan as a descending angel or, to use a storybook character, Mary Poppins. She must at least have seemed this way to the desperate Kellers, who had an out-of-control, deaf-blind child.

There is a scene in the movie that represents a professional climax. Shortly after arriving at the Kellers' home, Annie was to be introduced to her charge at a formal Sunday afternoon dinner. Annie was waiting at the fully laden table with Helen's father and brother. Mrs. Keller entered with Helen, and it was very apparent that she had no control over the child. Helen was making gruesome noises and totally disrupted the meal by throwing food. The father and brother left in a huff, and Mrs. Keller looked across the table to Annie in total despair.

At this point, Annie had a choice to make: to work with Mrs. Keller and teach her how to manage her child or to rescue Mrs. Keller by taking the child. If Annie had worked with Mrs. Keller, then Annie would not have become famous and would not have received the credit. Mrs. Keller might have! For Annie to have done this, she would have to have had what psychologists call an "inner locus of evaluation," the ability to pat oneself on the back and let others get the credit. To do this, one has to be a reasonably congruent person. Annie, given her deprived childhood and her very strong need to be needed, chose to take Helen to a shack on the property and literally strapped Helen to her at night. Within 2 weeks she emerged with a civilized child who was beginning to communicate—a miracle! Since most of the movie's viewers know that Helen turned out to be a truly remarkable deaf-blind person who achieved a great deal despite her disability, it is tempting to conclude that they lived happily ever after.

Lash's (1980) biography, however, continues the story. The effect of Annie's success on Mrs. Keller was profound. In a short time, Annie had accomplished more than Mrs. Keller had in the previous 6 years of trying to work with the child on her own. She was profoundly grateful, but at the same time more convinced than ever that she was an inadequate mother for such a child. After all, she could not work "miracles" the way Annie could. Mrs. Keller abandoned any further attempts to actively mother Helen and thereafter seemed to be reduced to the role of loving aunt.

Helen and Annie went back to Boston, and Helen achieved all the outward manifestations of success, including graduating from Radcliffe College. However, the closely dependent relationship that developed between them, in which Annie had almost all the control, could not work in Helen's (or in Annie's) best interest. The goal of teaching, like the goal of parenting, is to encourage the child to be independent. Annie could not do this with Helen because Annie had so many needs to be needed that had not been fulfilled in her life. In many ways, she needed Helen more than Helen needed her. After Annie's death, Helen went through a succession of paid companions, none of whom satisfied her in the way that Annie did. She never learned how to live independently despite her formidable and remarkable skills.

The Annie Sullivan story is an extreme example of the rescue syndrome. Sometimes the most helpful thing professionals can do for clients is to not help, or at least to not help in an overt manner. Often I have been much more useful to people who left my office saying, "Why did we go there? We knew all of that before we went," than to those who have left saying, "What would we ever do without him?" We work in a helping profession, but to be truly helpful, our goal must be to enhance our clients' and their families' self-esteem and thereby empower them. Overt assistance, although often appreciated, is also a statement that the recipient is inadequate and needs aid. Very often the overt aid leads to resentment on the recipient's part and also to diminished self-confidence. To nurture effectively is to give help in a sensitive, timely fashion that may not always be seen or appreciated by the recipient. We as professionals need to remain very much aware of our own needs to be needed, and to be able to pat ourselves on the back so that others may take the credit. Our goal in helping is to create independent people who no longer need help.

Anger

Almost anyone experiencing a catastrophic change will experience some anger. The person might not be aware of this anger and might not be able to express it, but it is there nonetheless. Anger has many sources, the predominant one being when there is a violation of expectations. At a very simple level, if I think you and I have an agreement to meet and you fail to show up, I will be angry. It is a self-righteous anger. All parents have many expectations about their unborn child, most significantly that he or she will be normal. When the child is "defective," the parents are angry; they feel cheated.

Another expectation, in many cases doomed to failure, is that the disorder can be cured. Parents find it harder to accept that there is no cure than to accept that the child has a disability. (They say, for example, "We spend so much money to send an astronaut to the moon; why can't we find a cure for cerebral palsy?") The clients also have expectations of the professional and usually expect to be taken care of à la Annie Sullivan. (They saw the movie The Miracle Worker, too.) This expectation may or may not be violated.

The most pervasive, and perhaps most harmful, expectation that clients have is the idealized image of how they should perform. This expectation is fed by a steady stream of sitcom families on TV who resolve crises easily and with apparent calmness. This sets up an expectation in clients and their families that they, too, should be able to manage the change with a minimum of stress and pain. When this is not the case, they feel angry at themselves for being so "incompetent" and "weak." They are not able to see the reality that they are quite normal. This self-directed anger is very harmful, often manifesting itself as depression and low self-esteem.

Dealing with or having a communication disorder causes a loss of some personal freedom, which becomes another source of anger. When disability is present, a client's and family's life options are narrowed and they get very angry at these restrictions. They have lost control of their lives. A father of a deaf child, for example, said,

I have been working for several years to get a promotion in my company. I have wanted this very badly and today I was informed that I have the promotion. If I take it, though, it means that we will have to move to a small town which has no services for the deaf, and my son will have to go to a school for the deaf on a residential basis. My wife and I consider this option terrible. So now if I take the promotion I will screw up my son, and if I don't I will damage my career. I am very angry and frustrated!

This father's anger is very typical, as is the frustration of many mothers who decide to stay home to take care of their disabled child and to forgo their career advancements. Spouses, too, must make adjustments in their life plans because of the disability of their husbands or wives. The corporate executive, for example, who can no longer function at meetings because of his progressive hearing loss will be very angry and resentful. His wife might also be angry at the restrictions in their social life and perhaps at being relegated to the role of, in the words of one wife, "a hearing ear dog." These are changes that are forced from the outside and over which people have little or no control. A loss of control always involves a great deal of anger.

Another source of anger, which is more like rage, is the parent's or spouse's frustration over having a loved one hurting in some way and the inability to make it better for the person. This feeling of impotence or powerlessness was devastating for me as I watched my wife stagger from one place to another and I was unable to make things better for her. All parents are pledged to make things better for their children; when they cannot, they feel a terrible impotence that manifests itself as rage. Fathers and husbands are more likely to experience this kind of anger because of their family role. Men traditionally are the family protectors. Their job is to stand at the gates and slay any dragons that might be assaulting the family. When family members are hurting, the father feels he has failed, and he becomes frustrated and angry. In women, the anger traditionally tends to be turned inward, becoming depression; in men, it usually gets displaced.

I think most professionals in our field recognize at some level that they are dealing with angry people. Many of the emotional distancing strategies employed—for example, keeping the relationship content based—are designed to keep at bay the eruption of the client volcano. Very often, client anger is displaced onto the professional, and the professional can easily become the lightning rod. People sometimes slay the messenger when they do not like the message.

Anger is a very difficult emotion in most relationships; it frequently is equated with loss of love. Most families do not have good strategies for dealing with anger other than to suppress it. It is usually seen as something very threatening to relationships and thus is often displaced onto innocent victims (dogs, cats, professionals) or turned inward to become depression.

When anger is subverted and not allowed to emerge, it poisons relationships. A person who is angry with me and does not tell me frequently operates in subversive ways. For example, the angry client chronically misses appointments, is bothered by very minor things such as the decor of the room or the comfort of the chair, and does not fully participate in the therapy. Unless I can tap into that anger and deal with it, the relationship will never be mutually satisfactory. If professionals do not deal well with their own anger, they become poor role models for their clients. Very often, professionals feel that they do not have the right to be angry with clients. How very demeaning this is to clients, because it also says, "You don't mean enough to me to provoke anger in me." Professionals will do many of the same things clients do in repressing and displacing their anger, thereby confounding the therapeutic relationship. Unexpressed anger in relationships is like a loaded cannon loose on deck that can go off at any moment and sink the vessel.

The source of much client–professional anger is implicit, unfulfilled expectations. In any relationship that has any degree of intimacy, the parties have expectations of themselves, of each other, and of the relationship. In a healthy relationship, almost all the expectations are made explicit so that if there is a violation of an explicit expectation, it can be dealt with in the course of the relationship. Less healthy relationships, and ultimately less stable ones, have many implicit expectations. These are the ones we assume the other person is going to fulfill, but we never express them to make them explicit. When these expectations are violated, we get angry; if we have not been explicit about our expectations, we cannot be direct about our anger, either.

For example, I may wake up in the morning wanting to have pasta for dinner, only I do not bother to tell my wife (I figure she loves me so much and we have been married long enough that she should be able to read my mind). So I go off to work expecting pasta for supper. When I return home, because my wife is not always accurate in her mind reading, I get something else for dinner, which under ordinary circumstances would be delicious, but I get angry because it is not pasta. (The reader will recognize here the Italy/Holland issue in another guise.) Because I know that I did not ask for pasta in the morning, I know I do not have a right to complain about the lack of pasta at night; that, however, does not stop me from feeling angry. Because I know I cannot be overt about the anger because it would not be fair, I wait for my wife to do something annoying that under ordinary circumstances I might ignore. If she drops and breaks a cup, for example, while I am carrying this load of unexpressed anger, I zap her, and we have a big fight about the broken cup when I am really angry about the pasta. As long as we continue to fight about the cup, our relationship makes no progress. Relationships can stand only so much of this before they crumble from the assaults of unfair anger. However, if we do argue about the pasta, we can renegotiate our contract and our relationship can become stronger for it.

Many professional–client relationships have failed because of implicit, unfulfilled expectations. Many expectations revolve, for example, around responsibility assumptions. A teacher may assume that the parent will be doing homework with the child, and the parent may assume that schoolwork is the province of the teacher. The undiscussed expectations lead to anger that is seldom expressed directly. The teacher and the parent need to discuss their mutual expectations and make a contract. Then if there is a failed expectation, the anger can be expressed directly and the contract renegotiated if necessary.

It is not the implicit expectations per se that create the problems (although it always helps to make explicit that which is implicit and see if there is a match on expectations); it is the unwillingness to be direct about the anger that defeats relationships. Anger can be a very healthy emotion in relationships. Because there is a great deal of caring and energy in anger, it becomes the fuel of change. If clients are angry at me, I examine the anger to see if it is justified. If I have been derelict in my duty, I apologize and make amends if possible. If we are dealing with a situation in which there has been an implicit expectation that I have failed to meet, the anger then becomes an opportunity to clarify our relationship and make the expectations explicit. If I am dealing with displaced anger, then we can clarify the anger. Very often, parents are angry at the child for having the disability. Because this anger is hard to acknowledge, it is easier for them to be angry at me, because I in some sense represent the disorder. I can clarify that they actually are angry at the situation in which they find themselves. This displaced anger very often can get rechanneled into more useful places, such as working to help other parents and children trying to live with the disability. Anger can be a very useful source of energy, especially if directed at politicians and bureaucrats who are inadequately funding programs.

There is never any loss in dealing openly and honestly with anger. It took me a long time to recognize that anger will not emerge unless there is a high degree of trust and intimacy in a relationship. Only secure people can afford to risk the loss of relationships by showing anger. Relationships are almost always strengthened after anger emerges if there is an acceptance of the feeling and a mutual willingness to explore the sources of the anger. The professional needs to be a secure person to allow client anger to emerge. If the groundwork has been laid in establishing trust, then the relationship can withstand and grow from controversy.

Guilt

I think that next to anger, guilt is the single most pervasive feeling experienced by the families of clients with disabilities. All parents, especially mothers, feel some guilt for a child who has a disability. I think guilt, in general, is more prevalent in the female population, reflecting the way girls are acculturated in our society. They are not allowed to feel powerful; rather, they are expected to be compliant and passive. Guilt becomes a power statement: It says that the individual has had some negative power to influence or cause this bad result. One mother in a parent group once said, "I even feel guilty when it rains." My response was, "Boy, you must be feeling very powerful, too." There is also power in worry. My mother-in-law, worrier par excellence, did this all the time; the implicit statement was that if she worried about an event, she could control it, and thus feel some sense of power.

Vulnerability

An existential fact of life is that we all are vulnerable. If we live long enough, something bad will happen to us, and if we don't live long enough, then something bad has already happened. To allay the anxiety caused by this fact of life, we develop a myth of invulnerability. We think bad things can't happen to us—they happen only to other people. To a large extent, we need this myth to function in our daily lives. Without it, we might never get into an airplane or drive a car; we might just spend our time cowering under the covers, and even then, we would not be safe. There is no safety in life. Nobody gets out of it alive.

When something bad does happen to us, such as having an autistic child, we feel that our cloak of invulnerability has been pierced. We realize how naked and alone we really are, and how fragile our existence is. We have lost the pseudo-comfort that the myth of invulnerability provided. This realization is scary and it may make us timid for a time. Parents undergoing a "crisis of vulnerability" seem very much like guilt-ridden, overprotective parents. A mother whose child was deafened by meningitis said,

> When I took her home from the hospital I wouldn't let her outside at all, and I wouldn't let any other children come in and play because I was afraid she

might get sick again. When I finally did take her with me to the supermarket, I brought along a can of disinfectant and sprayed the shopping cart. For the first year I lived in complete terror that she might get sick again.

The anxiety generated by the awareness of vulnerability, as opposed to the anxiety that is generated from unresolved guilt feelings, can be a positive force. When we recognize our vulnerabilities, we can and very often do reorder our priorities. We can live more fully as we recognize the finiteness of our existence. The mother of the child with meningitis also said,

> It made you more aware of things, more appreciative. It made me kind of stop and smell the flowers a lot more than I would before. I was always kind of rushing around and hurrying and not stopping as much as I do now. I'm just kind of enjoying everything as much as possible because you just realize, I don't know, maybe your vulnerability. Who knows what is going to happen next, so you might as well enjoy now. I used to think that that could never happen to me . . . but I don't feel that way anymore. Not in a real negative, pessimistic kind of thing, but it's life and you have no control over it, so you might as well appreciate what you have. Make the best of it.

That statement could have been written by any existential philosopher. If we allow parents to go through the grief process and we treat them with the loving respect they need, then all sorts of good things can happen to them. They can learn to take each day for the gift that it is, and although their life is not "Italy," "Holland" also has a lot to offer.

Confusion

Almost all of our clients, as they go through the learning process, experience confusion. Confusion is a normal, healthy part of the process of learning; as we attempt to acquire new information that we do not have the experience to evaluate, and a vocabulary that is totally unfamiliar to us, we are confused. In the resolution of the confusion, we learn, provided we are given time and repetition. Unfortunately, clients and their families, especially in the early stages of diagnosis, are given much more information than they can use. (See Chapter 1 for the effects of information counseling.) Professionals often use jargon and assume that after defining a term once or twice, the client has retained the meaning, which is usually not the case. We are often not aware of our jargon.

Terms such as *audiogram, audiologists,* and *decibel* are rather esoteric and unfamiliar to most people. I have found, for example, that parents of deaf children take about a year to understand an audiogram despite the many tests given to their children and the many explanations given by the audiologist. (At that, they are faster than some students in my beginning audiology class.)

Professionals are not the only source of "information" to clients. When someone has an apparent disability, he or she loses anonymity. The person can hardly walk outside without other people telling their inspirational stories and rendering advice. Walking with my wife in a wheelchair, for example, was an adventure. She got "God blessed" right and left, and people offered all kinds of free advice. If we weren't pretty secure in what we know, this avalanche of well-intended advice and information would bring us to despair rather than enlightenment. Information overload can be very harmful, because the increased confusion leads to increased feelings of inadequacy and anxiety, all of which tend to reduce self-confidence.

Professionals contribute to client confusion by providing information-based counseling when the client is not psychologically ready to receive it. In my early years, as an insecure professional, I used content counseling as the prime distancing strategy. If I focused a relationship on content (which also met both the client's and my expectations), then I could be in control and we did not need to tap into the feelings of grief and anger, with which I was very uncomfortable. This strategy severely limited the relationship, defining me as the source of knowledge, and extended the client's confusion and anxiety because I provided too much gratuitous information, too early in the grief process.

As professionals, we have a responsibility to provide information. As a general rule of thumb, I do not give clients information unless they ask for it. I generally ask, "What do you need to know?" When I receive a response such as, "I don't even know enough to ask a question!" which is fairly typical in the early stages, I might respond, "It sounds like you are pretty confused." This is an invitation to talk about client feelings. I have seen professionals who are anxious to get habilitation started tell parents who are too confused to ask questions, "Here are some things I think you need to know." This response must be resisted at all costs because it takes away client power and gives the professional too much responsibility. The content questions will emerge as the clients become more comfortable with their new status and are moved a bit further along in the grief process. If we facilitate the process by empathetic listening, the content will emerge.

When clients ask specific content questions, I answer them. I like to think that my answers are free of opinion, but I, like most professionals in the field, have strong biases. The best I can do is to identify my answers as opinions when talking with the parents. There is a need and a place for content, even in the early stages of relationships; it fulfills an implicit contract between professionals and their clients. I feel that information during the initial stages functions more to establish credibility than to alleviate ignorance. We must establish credibility to be truly helpful, but we also must remain sensitive to the relationship as it is being established.

These feelings—grief, anxiety, inadequacy, anger, guilt, vulnerability, and confusion—are turbulent and chaotic feelings that clients and their families experience when they encounter a disability in themselves or a family member. These people are emotionally upset, and very appropriately so. As was said at the outset of this chapter, feelings are neither good nor bad, and it is not our responsibility to make our clients feel better. We can, by our calm acceptance of their feelings and our willingness to allow feelings to be part of the client–professional relationship, prevent the development of secondary negative feelings. We can, for example, help to prevent clients from feeling guilty about their guilt feelings. When we do this, their coping process can begin. With our sensitive appreciation of the grief process, the clients' chaotic feelings can be transformed into positive behavior. Thus, the grief can become a sadness that also enables the clients to appreciate what they have, the anger can become the energy to make changes, the guilt can become commitment, the recognition of vulnerability can become the means by which clients reorder priorities, and the resolution of confusion can become the motivation for learning.

The Professional's Feelings

The feelings described in this chapter in relation to clients also characterize the professional's reactions. Nothing is abnormal or unhealthy about any of the feelings described. Under the skin we are all brothers and sisters. Audiologists, for example, often feel overwhelmed by and inadequate to cope with the responsibility of determining a child's hearing loss and of properly counseling the family. This is especially true of the beginning audiologist, who is still developing good test techniques and learning appropriate counseling strategies. Even veteran audiologists experience an anxiety almost akin to panic when presented with a child who promises to be difficult to test and a family that appears hard to counsel. Has any professional not felt the fear of that icy finger of failure? The anxiety becomes the spur for continued professional improvement.

Professionals also experience anger. They feel anger at parents for not following through on a recommended course of action; they feel rage, frustration, and sometimes despair when they can't make things better for the child or family with whom they are involved. They may feel intense anger at other professionals who insensitively or inappropriately treat the families, such as the pediatrician who fails to refer or the classroom teacher who doesn't understand the child's language difficulty. This anger provides the energy that can be used to educate other professionals and make programmatic changes. If repressed, it lends itself to depression and burnout.

Guilt is also a part of the professional's experience. I know of no responsible and competent speech and hearing professional who suffers no regrets about the handling of past cases. Mistakes—an inevitable part of the experience of all professionals—are our "nuggets of gold." They indicate to us what we need to learn next. All responsible professionals should be operating on their "fringes of incompetence." They should be taking risks and occasionally making mistakes, or they are not growing. Many speech and hearing professionals are needlessly burdened by the guilt associated with their risks. Fortunately, we are not brain surgeons. Almost all my clients have survived my mistakes quite well. Some have even flourished; so have I.

Those of us who work clinically, especially in hospital settings, are constantly confronted with people who have severe disorders. We are not given the luxury that most people have of retaining our myth of invulnerability. Daily we meet people like us who are in deep pain, and we often say, "There but for the grace of God go I." The recognition of our personal vulnerability can lead to our being very caring, thoughtful clinicians, and it can spill over into our personal lives, where we can reorder our priorities, much as our clients do when they realize what is really important in life.

Frequently when the feelings surrounding communication disorders are described, the negative and painful emotions are emphasized, while the positive feelings and experiences are seldom discussed. Often overlooked are the marvelous opportunities for joy and growth. Many parents come through the experience of having a hearing-impaired child with a clearer sense of themselves and of their priorities than they had before their child was diagnosed. Many parents discover that their child's disorder has given their life meaning and direction. Their joy stems from actively participating in their child's growth; they take nothing for granted. When their child reaches a milestone, they rejoice in the knowledge that they helped in the accomplishment. I am always reminded of the Bertrand Russell quote, "To be without some of the things you want is an indispensable part of happiness."

The speech and hearing professional also experiences joy in working with the families of clients. In the initial stages of diagnosis, everything appears bleak and hopeless to the families, and the speech pathologist or audiologist often becomes their lifeline. My most meaningful clinical experiences have been in the intimate relationships that I have had with parents of newly diagnosed hearing-impaired children. It is very gratifying to witness and participate actively in the process by which people grow and fulfill their potential. I often tell parents that I will share some of their pain if they will share some of their joy with me as well.

The Coping Process

In my research on chronic illness, I came across a coping process model that I have found very helpful in many of my clinical interactions. Again, the model is useful only as a guide, and the stages are not firmly fixed points as in climbing a mountain—once gained, never lost—but rather a fluid series of points in which even successfully coping individuals return to earlier stages. Matson and Brooks (1977), based on their interviews with patients who had multiple sclerosis, found four stages to the coping process: denial, resistance, affirmation, and integration. Let us look at these stages in relation to communication disorders.

Denial

Probably no single factor impairs client–professional relationships as much as the denial mechanism. Denial must be seen by the professional for what it is—namely, a coping strategy based on feelings of inadequacy; when a person is in denial, there is no psychological "owning" of the problem. The person may admit that the problem exists, but he or she is not emotionally engaged. Denial is a very normal, very human reaction that occurs in all of us.

When I am driving my car, for example, and the engine begins to sound strange, I respond by turning on the radio. If the engine noises get louder, I increase the volume. Although I know cognitively that turning on the radio is not going to solve my problem, at that time, psychologically, it is the only thing I can do. In short, I try to deny the existence of the problem, hoping that it will go away by itself. My need to adopt the radio strategy is based on my lack of confidence in my ability to repair engines. I feel totally inadequate around mechanical things, certainly anything as complicated as a car engine. If you were to admonish me about how silly I am to respond by turning on the radio, I would grin sheepishly and agree with you. At this point I use a passive-aggressive strategy that I learned as a child in how to deal with authority figures—that is, I agree with you and proceed to do what I was doing when you are not around. Unless I am given other ways of coping and gain some confidence in myself, I cannot afford to give up denial. If, for example, I successfully completed a course in engine maintenance with your help, then I might hear the slightest noise and pull the car to the side of the road because I feel I have some chance of solving the problem and I would therefore cope with the crisis in a more responsible way than by denying its existence.

Parents of a child with a disability begin to experience feelings of denial any time there is a new demand on parental resources, requiring that they be wise or strong. The most obvious time is at diagnosis: Often the delay in getting a child diagnosed is because the parents cannot admit to themselves that something may be wrong. Others in the parents' environment also practice denial, especially grandparents, and sometimes professionals such as the family pediatrician.

Denial persists even when the parents freely acknowledge that they have a child with a disability. In coping with deafness, denial occurs around anything that objectifies the deafness. The hearing aid, for example, becomes a powerful reminder of deafness. Parents may hate to see it on their child even though they know it helps. When they take pictures of the child, they remove the hearing aid. This, by the way, becomes a good measure of where the parents are on the coping model. Parents who are in the affirmation or integration stage insist that the hearing aid be worn, whereas those who are in the denial or resistance stage remove it for pictures. If the parents are in a total communication program, their denial can become focused on the signing; thus we have parents who never attend class or, when they do, cannot seem to learn how to sign.

The child-centered professional views parental denial as an impediment to the child's progress and gets angry at the parents. The professional who is direct about the anger gives the parents an admonitory lecture about how important it is for the child to wear the aid or how necessary it is for the parents to attend signing class. The parents agree with the professional; they knew how important it was before the professional told them, but because they have no other coping strategy—much as I didn't with my car—they fall back on denial. After an initial period of attendance at classes or increased hearing aid use, they often revert to denial, which provokes another round of professional ire. If not stopped, this negative parent–professional interaction can escalate to the point where there is no communication between parent and professional, to the detriment of the child.

The professional must learn to recognize the denial as a plea for help and not as a dereliction of duty on the parents' part. No parents, at least those whom I have met, want to do badly by their child, but their many fears get in the way of their operating constructively. The basis of denial is fear and ignorance abetted by low self-esteem. People cannot be urged out of denial. They give it up when they feel confident that they can be more successful with some other coping strategy. In general, it is best not to undermine the denial mechanism directly unless one has something better to offer in its stead. Giving up denial—the only way the clients feel that they can currently cope with the situation—with nothing to replace it would be overwhelming. The parents feel as if their psychological survival depends on denial, and in some respects it does. Denial is not given up easily. By listening and by indirect teaching, which does not diminish clients' feelings of competency, counselors can teach clients more fruitful coping strategies than denial.

If the professional is focused on the child and is anxious about the child's welfare, parental denial might provoke an adversarial relationship between the professional and the parents that can destroy any productive counseling relationship. Professionals often try to "save" the child from the parents. Short of removing the child from the home, this cannot be done. Children cannot be saved from their parents; all of us, in some sense, are victims of our parents' failings. The professional must not let parental denial impair the development of a healthy relationship. I don't think any successful counseling can take place unless the professional has some understanding of the denial mechanism.

The identification of behavior as denial can be very tricky. It is not always clear when the clients are denying or when there is a legitimate difference of opinion between the client and the professional. Labeling can be used to try to substitute professional "truth" for parental "truth"—and room must be allowed for a difference of opinion.

One person's denial may be another person's optimism. Frequently, when the professional has a very pessimistic prognosis for a child, the parent keeps saying, "He will make it." Children have a way of meeting expectations, and when the expectations are negative, children seldom perform well. I have often seen the parents proved right; there is never any need to diminish parental optimism as long as their behavior is consistent with accepted management practices. The optimism frequently gets translated into hope, and many parents have the "maybe someday they will find a cure" dream. This dream, which enables them to work vigorously in the present and sustains them when they despair, should never be doused by the professional. There is probably no crueler act than to deprive the parents of this dream.

There is also much that is positive about denial. In 1962, the U.S. government declared all Spanish–American War veterans, of which there were only several hundred in the United States, totally disabled. This declaration, which entitled them to receive full benefits at the Veterans Administration, occasioned the launching of a large-scale study of the aged male. These men were in their 80s at the time, and the study involved gathering data on all aspects of their lives. I was involved in studying their hearing. As part of the examination, I interviewed them about how well they thought they could hear. This part of the research protocol became meaningless, as every one of them felt he could hear fine, despite the fact that in many instances I had to shout to be heard. I spoke to the project psychologist about this phenomenon, and he said it was pervasive throughout the study. These men persistently denied any infirmity, and he concluded—only partially tongue in cheek—that perhaps one of the major secrets of living to a ripe old age is to assiduously practice denial.

Resistance

Denial blends into resistance and at times is indistinguishable from it. In the resistance stage, the client and the family say, "We have a problem here but we are going to be a special case. We will somehow prevail over the disorder." Parents of a deaf child, for instance, say, "I know he is deaf but he is going to be a super deaf person. He will have normal speech, be a marvelous lip reader, and have an amazing job that few people will ever expect a deaf person to have." My first wife, shortly after being diagnosed as having multiple sclerosis, ran a 10-k race as though to defiantly say, "Being a cripple won't happen to me." As I watched her stagger across the finish line, I was filled with both admiration and anxiety for her. That was the last race she ever ran.

Resistance differs from denial in that the persons acknowledge to themselves that they have a problem and they work very hard to defeat it. In resistance, there is almost always a private pledge to conquer the disorder, as well as a rejection of help from any organizations that deal with the disorder. During the resistance stage, clients are unwilling to join any support groups or receive help in the form of meeting with peer counselors. They are in effect "closet" disabled. In the early stages of diagnosis, my wife and I did not, for example, want to meet anyone who had multiple sclerosis. For years, I found it very hard, if not impossible, to go to meetings where there were adults who were severely disabled by the condition. I just didn't want to be reminded of my potential future. (My wife was much better at this than me.)

In resistance, a great deal of energy is directed almost frantically and secretly at proving that the professionals are "wrong." Both denial and resistance are used to forestall or minimize the pain of the grief process. In denial, one says, "I don't really have this problem." In resistance, the person says, "I will lick this problem."

The difficulty for clients and their families comes about when they realize that they have a disorder that they cannot defeat. For parents of a deaf child, this sometimes happens as late as the child's adolescence, when they realize that he or she is not going to be the super deaf adult that they had expected; another dream dies and the grief process starts anew.

Clients often need to hit an emotional bottom in order to move on with the coping process. They need to see for themselves that denial does not work and that frantic resistance is not productive before they can mourn deeply their loss and move into the affirmation stage. To move to that stage, they need to have some confidence in their own ability to cope with the disorder in a proactive manner.

Affirmation

In the affirmation stage, the loss is acknowledged both to the self and to the world at large. Affirmation is a statement that "I am now a different person, and our family is also different." During this stage of coping, the family is consumed by the disorder. Energy is devoted toward ameliorating the effects of the disorder. In this stage, families become very active in organizations designed to educate the members and the public at large. One such group, SHHH (Self Help for Hard of Hearing People), is designed as a support/educational group for people who are hard of hearing. In groups such as SHHH, members get an opportunity to establish their new identity as "hard-of-hearing persons"; they have come out of the disability closet. The new identity may be taken on tentatively or proudly (as we have seen in the deaf community), but it is a public acknowledgment of the new identity. In this stage, an intense desire to help others arises. One parent of a deaf child said, "When you first find out your child is deaf, you feel badly for yourself. After a while you feel badly for your child. Now I feel badly for all deaf children." This movement outside of one's own pain is very healthy and marks the transition into integration.

Integration

Integration (also known as acceptance) is characterized by getting the disorder into a life perspective. The client and family learn to live with the disorder and to spend time and energy on other matters. The client is able to say, "I am more than a walking hearing disorder; I am a person who does not hear well, but many other aspects of my life need to be developed." In the integration stage, although there is still pain for the loss, and at times grief, the changes caused by the disorder are integrated into a new lifestyle with different values. The affirmation and integration stages are reached when the individual realizes that "beating" the disorder is not always a matter of reaching normalcy, but rather of learning to live life to the fullest in the face of the disorder.

Individuals vary as to the degree and speed with which they can get to integration. Some families seem forever stuck in denial, which seems to them to be the only possible coping strategy; they are paralyzed in their fear. Others move through the process very rapidly, seeming to skip stages. The key is the self-confidence of the families. When they feel secure in their abilities to cope, it becomes easier to assume the psychological risk of giving up the pseudo-comfort of denial and resistance to assume the responsibilities demanded by the affirmation and integration stages of the coping process. Let us look now specifically at coping.

All coping involves a stressful interaction between a person and the environment. Coping is any response to a difficult life situation that avoids or prevents distress. Successful coping always involves the possibility of growth and always demands change. It is the people who are uncomfortable who will grow because they are forced to derive a new set of responses to contend with a changing set of either internal or external demands. We tend to give to life what life demands of us, and when we are stressed by an external force, we must find within us the strength and develop within us the resources to cope successfully. Coping is a dynamic process; it is not a stage finally won and held forever. At times it is a moment-to-moment proposition.

Pearlin and Schooler (1978), in a definitive article on coping, outlined four strategies that individuals use to cope with very difficult situations: flight, modification, reframing, and stress reduction.

Flight

The first and perhaps primary coping strategy is flight. Each person, when confronted with a difficult and potentially stressful situation, must decide whether to fight or take flight. In some situations in life, a person feels ill equipped to survive and decides that his or her own personal or psychological survival depends on removal from the situation. This may not be the reality of the situation, but as long as people feel that they cannot cope successfully, then flight will occur. It is the person's perception of events that is critical.

Many divorces occur in families with children with disabilities, and estrangements are common in families with adults with disabilities. Sometimes an adult child leaves a parent to struggle alone with a spouse with a disability. As a coping strategy, flight always leaves the person vulnerable to guilt and loss of self-esteem. In addition to the actual flight, as in a divorce, there is the psychological flight that occurs very frequently in parents and spouses of family members with disabilities. The psychological flight often takes the form of a fantasy about the death of the child or spouse. This is a deep-seated "wish" that is difficult for many parents or spouses to admit because they feel enormously guilty about having these feelings. When they do admit these fantasies to a professional, there usually is a high degree of trust in the relationship and they expect the professional to accept their statement at face value. It is critical that the professional accept this admission in a matter-of-fact manner. These feelings are very common. I often tell parents and spouses that I don't think they are wishing their child or spouse dead, but that they are wishing that this situation, which is so stressful to them, would go away.

Death fantasies may be helpful in preparing for the actual death of a spouse. This anticipatory mourning is seen frequently in spouses of clients with aphasia and in families in which someone has traumatic head injuries. Anticipatory mourning, which helps the person make the adjustment to living without the person with a disability, is part of the psychologically protective transition process that eases the way into an anticipated new status. The person is trying on the new role, which is very helpful, although it generally causes the person to feel a great deal of guilt. Professionals must never judge these fantasies, which almost always serve a useful psychological function as long as they remain fantasies.

Modification

If a person decides to stay with the family member with a disability, then the next strategy employed is to modify the situation. Stress can be reduced by direct intervention that reduces or modifies the disability. The client who gets a hearing aid and the patient with aphasia who gets a wheelchair and language therapy may reduce the stress caused by their losses. All therapy administered by a speech and hearing clinician is designed to reduce stress and help clients and their families cope better with communication situations.

Unfortunately, in our field there are many situations in which the stress of a disorder can be modified but not eliminated. For example, even with the best amplification, many clients will still have a significant hearing loss. We must help these clients to accept their limitations and to recognize that they cannot modify their environment any further. The trick in trying to modify the stressful situation is to know what can be modified and do it, and then learn to accept what cannot be changed—not always easy to do.

Reframing

Because the cognitive process always determines the emotional intensity of any event, for those elements of a situation that cannot be modified, stress can be reduced by changing the way a person views the situation. This is known as *reframing* or *cognitively neutralizing* the stressor. The most commonly used cognitive neutralizer is the phrase, "It could be worse," whereupon parents or spouses proceed to mention someone, someplace who is in more difficulty than they are in ("He could have cancer," "He could be deafer," "He could have died," etc.). This is known as a "positive comparison." The problem with using positive comparisons as a reframing strategy is that there are still times when the client or the family member feels upset about the disability. When this happens, they usually feel guilty because they feel they have forfeited their right to grieve. My wife's response to "It could be worse," was to say, "Yes and it could be better, too!"

Using positive comparisons often buys some short-term relief, but the disability will always intrude, and the effectiveness of looking for someone worse off begins to fade quickly. There are other more fruitful ways of reframing, which are discussed in Chapter 6.

Stress Reduction

The fourth strategy is to deal directly with the stress. No matter how successful modification and reframing might be, many clients will still experience stress with which they must learn to live. Each individual must find his or her own individual stress reducers, and what is effective for one person may not work for another. In my interviews with the spouses of patients with chronic illness, I found that exercise and work are almost universal stress reducers. Exercise is effective in part because it is a timeout experience that gets the well spouse away from confronting the spouse with a disability. It also is an emotionally calming activity; exercise, especially repetitive exercise, such as jogging, swimming, or bicycling, seems to put the mind into a meditative state. Work serves as a distraction. Well spouses can immerse themselves in problems that have solutions and are controllable. They also are in contact with other adults with whom they can talk and think about something other than their spouses. In fact, one of my definitions of a "shadow spouse" is someone who looks forward to going to work and dreads coming home.

When speech and hearing professionals encounter clients, the traumatic events have already happened, and the grief and coping processes are already under way. By virtue of the way we interact with clients and their families, we can facilitate or retard the coping process. This is especially true at the diagnostic evaluation, which is usually close to the time of the catastrophic event. When clients' feelings are very fluid and apparent because the impact of the disorder has not settled in yet, we can alter very dramatically the course of the coping and the habilitation of the client.

COUNSELING AND THE DIAGNOSTIC PROCESS

The diagnostic interaction is critical for determining the future course of the client–professional relationship. It is the first step on a long journey for many clients, and it is an imprinting process that sets up in the client's mind future expectations of professional behavior. If the initial client–professional interaction has a feeling component and if clients are empowered at the outset, then they will expect and perhaps demand empowerment and affect in future contacts with professionals. Unfortunately, because of the prevalence of the medical model, the professional's role is usually restricted to providing information and prescribing what the client should do. In this model, the client is encouraged to become a passive participant in the habilitation program by simply "following the doctor's orders." In this chapter, I contrast institution-centered diagnosis and client-centered collaborative diagnosis.

Institution-Centered Diagnosis

In the medical model, a careful case history is obtained and tests are given. If a child is being tested, he or she is separated from the parents while the professional administers the tests. (If the parent is allowed to be present, it is usually as a passive observer.) After the testing, the professional "counsels" the parents by giving the test results and recommending what the parents should do next. As a beginning audiologist, I found the medical model very helpful. I soon developed some set speeches that I could give at the end of testing a child. They were similar to "tapes" I could plug in, for example, to describe how hearing aids worked; to explain audiograms; and, for parents of newly diagnosed deaf children, to provide a list of schools for the deaf in the area and describe the various educational methodologies used in the schools. On the surface, the medical model seems very efficient. Because I could control the interaction time, I could block out a prescribed time and see the maximum number of cases in a given day. I could fit each speech into a 10- or 15-minute period and then send the parents on their way; I felt that I had fulfilled my clinical obligation and, perhaps as important, I could see my next patient on time. I also succeeded in limiting the affective exchange so that I did not have to deal with feelings, about which I felt very insecure. After a while I stopped "seeing" patients; the visits simply became very routine and mechanical for me.

A variation of the individual medical model is the diagnosis-by-committee process, which on the surface is even more efficient. Many hospitals and educational programs operate this way when they have, for example, an Individualized Education Program (IEP). In this model, the child is tested by an array of professionals, usually on the same day, but sometimes spread over 2 or 3 days. The parents are then invited to a conference at which each professional delivers his or her report. Professionals in these meetings seldom talk directly to the parents. They are so busy trying to impress everyone else with their competency that they are speaking to impress rather then express; jargon abounds. Parents are glassy-eyed and generally traumatized by the whole experience. Imagine the experience from the parents' perspective of having a group of "experts" sitting around a table telling you what is wrong with your child. It has to be a nightmare!

Currently at Emerson College, research is under way in which parents who have undergone the diagnosis-by-committee process are interviewed. They report that they retained almost none of the material presented to them. They report feeling very scared and very numb. We have yet to find any parents who liked or appreciated the experience. At best, they found it helpful "because they didn't have to make so many trips to the hospital." All found it psychologically painful.

My personal opinion is that diagnosis by committee should be banned by the Geneva Convention as cruel and unusual punishment. It is used because it seems efficient to be able in one fell swoop to have the complete diagnosis. The efficiency is only illusory, however. Diagnosis by committee is convenient for the institution or the professionals; it is not efficient when one examines its effects on the families. Instead of retaining much of what is said, they remember unimportant details, such as the color of the doctor's tie or the kind of glasses he or she wore. They always remember the date vividly, and can describe the trip to the hospital in explicit detail, but they usually fail to retain any of the important information (Martin, Krueger, & Bernstein, 1990).

Any diagnostic process can only be as good as the counseling techniques and procedures employed. Of what use is it to have highly accurate tests and highly "efficient" procedures if professionals cannot communicate them effectively to the clients? The data we have indicate that the medical model is not an effective tool, whether it is by committee or by individuals. The research cited in Chapter 1 (Lerner, 1988; Martin et al., 1990; Williams & Derbyshire, 1982) shows how little parents retain of the information provided and how little they trust the audiologist. There are much better ways to conduct a diagnostic examination, which, although it may involve more time in the initial stages, will be much more efficient in the long term. The recommended approach is a client-centered collaborative model, as opposed to the institution-centered approach of the medical model.

Client-Centered Collaborative Diagnosis

There are two diagnostic scenarios: a deferred diagnosis and a congenital or sudden inception. In the deferred diagnosis, the child can be born with a disability, but the parents are unaware of the disability's existence and they leave the hospital thinking they have a normally developing child. The realization that something is wrong with the child will usually occur over time, and the diagnostic process will then be parent driven. On the other hand, with a congenital disability, which is apparent at birth, or a sudden onset of a disability, the diagnostic process will be institution driven and begins at birth or the inception of the disability.

Deferred Diagnosis

Let us look first at the deferred diagnostic process when the disability is not apparent at birth. For a good diagnostic examination, it is important that the professional understand and have some empathy for the client's history. When clients are first seen in the clinic, they bring with them a long history of their personal struggles with the realization that something is wrong. For example, a scenario for the parents of a child with a language learning delay might be something like this: One parent, usually the mother, becomes aware that something is wrong with the child. The first fear that parents frequently have when they suspect something is wrong is that their child might have mental retardation. (Retardation is generally what parents fear most and are most likely to fixate on.) When the mother begins to localize problems in the lack of speech and understanding, she confides her fears to the father, who responds by denying it, reassuring his wife and himself that nothing is wrong with their baby, and commenting that he or some member of his family spoke late and is subsequently fine (grandparents are notorious for also using this excuse). At this point, each parent embarks on a surreptitious program of testing the child's language comprehension without confiding his or her fears to the other. Now the parents are on an emotional roller coaster; they are elated when they get a response or a pseudoresponse, and crushed when the child fails to respond.

The denial mechanism is activated very early during this deferred diagnosis process, and parents tend to find many reasons as to why their child does not respond. (This is equally true for any insidious neurological disease. My first wife and I, for example, spent a great deal of time at the inception of the disease explaining away her vague neurological symptoms; one becomes an expert at finding benign reasons for frighteningly deviant behavior.) This period of uncertainty is very painful as the individuals vacillate between the peaks of relief and the valleys of fear and anxiety. Finally, the denial mechanism, battered by the assault of accumulated data, gives way, and with a great deal of trepidation, the families approach a professional for a diagnosis of the disorder. At this point, the families have generally agreed that something is wrong; they sustain themselves with the thought that medical science will be able to cure the disorder. They think that if their child has a language delay, an operation or a device will enable the child to speak again. (My wife and I hoped that the neurologist would be able to recommend a drug or a course of action that would cure the disorder or at least prevent further decline in her functioning. I remember also hoping that he would simply attribute her symptoms to increasing age.) All clients come to this diagnostic situation with the fear that there is something wrong but also with some sustaining hope that their fear is groundless and they will be proved wrong or that the disorder is readily amenable to a cure. It is the dashing of this hope that is so painful and that initiates the grief reaction.

Clients are always very anxious when they arrive at the clinic. They do not know what to expect; they are hoping against hope that they are wrong. They have composed a story detailing their experiences to date and they need to be allowed a chance to tell it to someone who will listen to them. That is why it is essential that they be given a chance to tell their story. A question such as, "Can you tell me what brought you here?" will generally elicit the story.

Client-centered counseling in the diagnostic process begins at the moment of the initial contact with the family and is continuous throughout the relationship. At the outset, the counselor needs to establish the families' major concerns and their expectations of the professional. Typically families express some concern about their family member's hearing or speech (although one can get very surprising answers to the question, "What concerns you most about your child?"). I don't try at this point to get a case history from the families; I simply let them tell me anything that they think is important. Later I will get to the more specific details.

After the family has shared their concerns and told their story, I enlist them as coworkers. I say something to them like, "I may be an expert on the testing of speech and language, but you are certainly an expert on this child; I need your help."

This remark about needing help is not a ploy to get parents involved but is very much the truth. Parents have a great deal of information about the child that can be used in the diagnostic process. Parents can come to the testing with most of the information in hand. Dale (1991) found that parents' self-reports of vocabulary and syntax of 2-year-old children correlated .79 with the standardized tests administered to the children. He strongly recommended that parents' self-reports be utilized in speech and language evaluations because they are

1. more representative of infant and toddler language than laboratory samples;

2. cost-effective for a rapid general evaluation of child language;

3. helpful in selecting assessment procedures for more in-depth analyses, if they are used before the child is seen; and

4. useful for monitoring changes that may result from intervention.

But above all else, the self-report, which enlists the parents as codiagnosticians, begins the process of empowering the parents. When I am conducting the audiological examination, I also bring in any other family members who have accompanied the parents, including grandparents and siblings. If it gets too chaotic, I may ask the other family members to leave. Often, though, they are very helpful, especially an older sibling, whom I generally use to condition the child being diagnosed, as described later. I proceed to start testing the child, usually giving one parent the audiogram to fill out. In this way the information that they need is being incorporated into what they are doing and seeing. The audiogram becomes much more meaningful to them because they are using it. When I am testing an adult, I usually have a family member in the test module with me, filling in the audiogram and scoring the discrimination tests. At the time an appointment is made for the examination, it is strongly suggested that the adult with a hearing impairment be accompanied by a family member.

When a sound comes on, I describe how loud the test sound is in terms of decibels and in terms of environmental stimuli (e.g., "This sound is about as loud as people talking"). Then I ask the parents whether they thought their child heard the sound. Depending on the age of the child, we might use visual reinforcement audiometry, where a light is paired with a sound, or play audiometry, where the child is conditioned to respond to a particular sound, for example, by placing a block in a toy mailbox. If the parents and I disagree as to whether the child heard the sound, I present the sound again until we have some agreement. At the end of the testing, I ask the parents what they think about their child's hearing, and we decide whether the child has a hearing loss. If we cannot agree, we continue testing, or if the child is not cooperative, we schedule another appointment with the Scotch verdict of "not proven." I never overrule the parents' opinion. Although I might hold to my opinion that the child does have a hearing loss, I never impose it on the parents; they would lose too much power if I did this and would not be fully invested in the child's habilitation program.

Parents have recounted to me years later their feelings during this kind of testing process. They frequently report how painful it was to sit in the room and hear those loud sounds while their child showed no response. This procedure diminishes the denial mechanism because the parents actually witness the hearing impairment. There is no way out for them because the testing procedure is modified according to their perceptions, and they are the ones who actually do the diagnosis.

Clinical procedures that separate the families from the testing process frequently increase denial because the parents can fantasize about the testing; that is, they can speculate that maybe the machine was broken or tracings were switched or any number of explanations caused the results. Although procedures that separate the parents and child might be more clinically accurate in detecting and determining the disability because there are no distractions for the tester, they are worthless if the parents cannot or will not accept the results. Parents have a need to "view the body." There is tremendous folk wisdom in the traditional funeral ritual when people go to the funeral parlor and view a body in the open casket, and then accompany the hearse to the cemetery and watch the casket lowered into the open grave. At first this might seem cruel, but it is psychologically very sound because it diminishes the denial reaction and allows the grief process to begin. The needed restructuring of one's life because of the loss can then commence. Among the more psychologically disabled people in our society have been the families of Vietnam War veterans who are still missing in action. These families cannot commit fully to a new life because they have not participated in a funeral and have no sense of closure. There is always a part of them that expects their loved ones to return, and they can imagine all sorts of scenarios in which they still might be alive. Denial in this case forestalls grief and delays or diminishes the necessary life restructuring.

Active parental involvement in the diagnostic process not only diminishes the denial mechanism, but also strengthens the bond between the clinician and the parents. Parents have reported to me how glad they were that I was helping them through the painful process. I was seen as an ally rather than an adversary. Audiologists and speech-language pathologists who deliver the word to parents in the waiting room that their child is impaired, no matter how nicely they do it, are often received with hostility; people often "kill the messenger when they don't like the message." Tattersall and Young (2006) found, in their study of parents whose children where identified as deaf in the newborn screening program in England, that parental satisfaction with the testing process was a function of when parents were enabled to feel partners in the process, and the program invited them to be active participants, not passive observers of what was occurring.

Another benefit of having the parents as codiagnosticians is that they are also being educated about the testing process. The information is gradually delivered to them and, because they are participating, it is retained much more readily than when a professional delivers a rote speech at the end of the testing to parents who have been sitting in the waiting room. Participating parents not only understand the test results better, but also obtain an idea of what their child can and cannot comprehend in the home environment, information that becomes very useful for them in the habilitation process. Participating in this way is especially helpful for the families of adults because it lets them see the extent of the disability and enables them to effectively participate in the rehabilitation process.

If we decide, after completing the testing, that the child is hearing impaired, I do not supply gratuitous information. Although I know that parents "need" a lot more information to effectively manage their child's habilitation than I give on that first session, I also know that at this point I can't overwhelm them with information. At this time I ask the parents, "What do you need to know now?" or "How can I be helpful to you now?" These questions at the end of the diagnostic tests are empowering because they allow the client and family to guide their own learning experience. I usually get a few desultory questions, which I answer simply because I know that the parents are in a state of shock. Parents have often told me that after the definitive diagnosis, all they wanted to do was go someplace and cry. Sometimes the parents with a deferred diagnosis actually respond to the diagnosis with relief, first because it is deafness and not retardation, of which they were mortally afraid, and second because somebody finally believed them and gave a name to the deviant behaviors of their child. With a name for the disorder, people sometimes think there is a way of controlling it. It is the information that there is no cure for the deafness that begins the grief process.

I have found over the years that one cannot go any faster with a child than the parents are willing or able to go. Clinicians limit truly effective case management when they become overwhelmed by their own anxiety to get the habilitation process moving. They then try to bypass the parental grief reaction by taking very active management of the case, leading invariably to passive, dependent parents and to ineffective tong-term management of the child. I feel very strongly that if we pay careful attention to the family members during the early stages of the diagnostic process, by taking time for them and giving them space to grieve, then the child or the identified adult client will do well in the long term. This may require the professional to sometimes let time elapse between the diagnosis and the initiation of habilitation procedures. It is difficult for most professionals, however, to see a child needing service and not getting it immediately.

I came across the following poem, written by Janice Fialka, a professional who is also a parent, that captures the essence of the interpersonal, affective dimension of the diagnostic process.

Advice to Professionals Who Must Conference Cases

Before the case conference,
I would look at my almost five-year-old son
And see a golden hair boy
Who giggled at his new baby sister's attempt to clap her hands,
Who charmed adults by his spontaneous hugs and hello's,
Who captured his parents with his rapture with music and his care for white haired people who walked a walk a bit slower than younger folks,
Who often became a legend in places visited because of his exquisite ability to befriend a few special souls,
Who often wanted to play "peace marches,"
And who, at the age of four,
went to the Detroit Public Library
requesting a book on Martin Luther King.

After the case conference,
I looked at my almost five-year-old son.
He seemed to have lost his golden hair.
I saw only words plastered on his face.
Words that drowned us in fear and revolting nausea.
Words like:
Primary expressive speech and language disorder
severe visual motor delay
sensory integration dysfunction
fine and gross motor delay
developmental dyspraxia and
RITALIN now.

I want my son back. That's all.
I want him back now. Then I'll get on with my life.
If you could feel the depth of this wrenching pain.
If you could see the depth of our sadness
then you would be moved to return
Our almost five-year-old son
who sparkles in the sunlight despite
his faulty neurons.

Please give me back my son
undamaged and
Untouched by your labels, test results,
descriptions and categories.

If you can't
If you truly cannot give us back our son

Then
just be with us quietly,
gently,
and compassionately as we feel.

Just sit patiently
and attentively as
we grieve and feel powerless.

Sit with us and create a stillness known only in small, empty
chapels at sundown.
Be there
With us as our witness and as our friend.

Please do not give us
advice,
suggestions,
comparisons or
another appointment. (That's for later.)

We want only
a quiet shoulder
upon which to rest our too-heavy heads.

If you can't give us back our sweet dream
then
comfort us through this nightmare.

Hold us.
Rock us
until morning light creeps in.

Then we will rise
and begin the work of a new day.

—Janice Fialka, MSW, ACSW
(Copyright 1994 by the author. Reprinted with permission.)

Another question I ask parents when we emerge from the test booth is, "Can you share with me how you are feeling?" This is an invitation to talk about affect. I sometimes give parents a bit of help by saying, "Some parents at this time feel like they have been hit by a truck," or maybe, "Some parents feel like they are walking through someone else's nightmare." Occasionally, parents begin to cry, and I stay with them. My own experience has led me to believe that the parents who cry most at the initial diagnostic session do better long term than those parents who seem to accept the diagnosis stoically. The "criers" are usually not very adept at using denial, and they are taking emotional ownership of the disability quickly. After the initial falling apart, they usually recover quite well and get readily to work. The "stoics" very often are buttressed by denial and sometimes never make it out of denial to work effectively with their child.

A frequent mistake that audiologists make with parents of a child who has a relatively mild hearing loss is to try to cheer up the parents by saying it could be much worse. First, it is always a mistake to try to cheer up people in pain because doing so invalidates their feelings. The message received is that they have no right to feel badly. Second, the degree of disability is always in the eyes of the beholder. To these parents, the disorder is very severe, and their feelings need to be respected and not minimized. At this point, the parents need someone to listen to them nonjudgmentally, someone who is not trying to focus their attention on content that they cannot absorb.

At the end of the first meeting, I give parents of newly diagnosed children the name and phone number of parents of an older child with a hearing impairment (they seldom call at first, as they are still in denial), and I set up an appointment to see them again within a week. I may reframe the situation for parents by saying that this diagnosis has guaranteed them an interesting life—not the one they thought they were going to have, but an interesting one nonetheless. In subsequent appointments I supply more information as the parents ask for it and seem ready to receive it. I start each session with that same question, "What do you need to know now?" or "How can I be helpful to you?" I have found that the parents eventually ask all the important questions.

The questions might not be in the same order that would occur if I were in complete control of the content, but the important issues are covered. Parents ask each question when they are ready for the answer. Although it may take a bit longer to get the hearing aid on the child or to have the child enrolled in an educational program than if I had taken initial control, he or she will get there nonetheless. What is important is that the child gets there with parents who have taken responsibility and have actively participated in the educational decisions and are, therefore, more likely to follow through on good educational management practices.

Speech-language pathologists can conduct diagnostic evaluations of children in the same way. For example, in a speech or language evaluation, parents can be enlisted as codiagnosticians and experts on their child's behavior, and they can score the test results or elicit responses from the child. This empowers as well as educates the parents. For adult patients, it is necessary to empower the spouse (or significant other) as well as the client. I always bring spouses into the audiometric test booth and sometimes have them give the hearing test or mark the audiogram. Clients always select their own hearing aids and guide all aspects of their testing. Rollins (1988) recommended conducting examinations of aphasic patients with the spouse as the active tester and the speech-language pathologist as the "coach." The job of counseling becomes much easier when the family participates actively in obtaining the diagnostic information.

One question that emerges very quickly, once the diagnosis is agreed upon, is the cause of the disorder. Handling this question is a very delicate counseling issue. One must determine responsibility without affixing blame. Parents who are obsessed with finding the cause are usually obsessed with guilt. They are looking to find a "cause" that is not their guilty secret. Each parent may be looking to blame the spouse or anyone else. It is very tricky handling this situation, and the careful clinician must steer a course between the Scylla of blame and the Charybdis of uncertainty. For a successful outcome, parents must give up the past and the search for the cause and deal constructively with their "now." It is often fruitful to begin to explore the guilt issue at this time, although it may be hard to elicit. I have found that a rather neutral statement, such as, "It must be so easy to feel guilty when you have had responsibility for bearing the child for so long," can be helpful to the mother, who is pressing me to find a cause for her child's deafness. I sometimes may ask her if she thinks she might have done something to cause her child to be deaf. This requires a great deal of sensitivity and trust and will be discussed more in the next chapter. I also tell her that she may have to learn to live with uncertainty as she may never know for sure what caused the child's deafness.

I often meet parents who don't seem to react at all to the diagnosis. In families in which a great many negative things have happened, the deafness is just one more thing. For example, a mother with three children came to our clinic. Her husband had left the family homeless and penniless. The mother had minimal physical and emotional energy to deal with her daughter's deafness. When told of the hearing loss, she responded with resignation.

People display their feelings in different ways. Some families and some cultures feel that it is inappropriate to display feelings publicly. These families seem to not react to the diagnosis although they may be deeply pained. Clinicians must not project themselves onto parents and expect all families to respond in the way they themselves would if they had just found out that their children were impaired. It is very easy to become judgmental about families; however, this must be avoided at all costs.

I see the diagnostic occasion as the first step on the long journey that many clients have before them. If we as professionals do our job well, we can make that a giant step and help the clients avoid many pitfalls that await them. We can also make it much easier for the professionals who are further down the clients' habilitation road.

To summarize, there are seven steps needed for a healthy, client-centered, collaborative diagnostic process:

1. Allow the client and family to tell their story. An open-ended question such as, "What brought you here?" is usually very helpful.

2. Enlist the family as codiagnosticians. Empower them with a statement such as, "You are the expert on this child, and I'll be the expert on the testing."

3. Involve the family and client actively in the testing procedure. The client should have choices where possible, and the family can be active in eliciting or scoring responses.

4. Have the client and family participate fully in the final diagnosis. In an ideal situation, they will make the diagnosis.

5. Empower them by asking, "What do you need to know now?" or "How can I be helpful to you?" Let them guide you as to how much information you should give.

6. Listen and respond to the family's affect. Give clients a chance to talk about how they feel in an unhurried, caring atmosphere. If there is a time limit, then tell the family this at the outset, for example, "I have 15 minutes before my next appointment; how can I be helpful to you?"

7. Set up another appointment. Do not try to cover everything in one

appointment. If this is not possible, help the family locate additional support in the form of peer counseling.

Congenital or Sudden Inception

The congenital or sudden diagnosis, as with an adult who has had a stroke, presents a somewhat different scenario and problem for the professional. This situation results in an institution-driven diagnosis given to generally unsuspecting family members. This scenario results when the child is born with a cleft palate or Down syndrome, or is diagnosed with a hearing loss following newborn screening. Newborn hearing screening has changed the diagnostic paradigm for deafness from deferred to congenital in many cases. The sudden-onset diagnostic is cataclysmic for the family, as there is no preparation and the shock is usually profound. In this paradigm, there is a limited case history per se, but the family members will be strongly invested in examining the past to find a cause. Family members are usually overwhelmed with the enormity of the situation, very much frightened and in a state of shock. It is especially fruitless to give much information in the initial stages of the sudden diagnosis. Responses that help elicit their feelings, which will be discussed in the next chapter, are usually most helpful at this time. Family members often need an opportunity to vent their feelings before they can get to a cognitive understanding of their situation. They need time, compassion, and above all else someone to listen to them. They will frequently tell the same story over and over again until it becomes their reality. They will be slow to ask information-seeking questions, but when they do, the professional needs to provide honest answers that are tuned to the family's level of understanding.

In the congenital diagnosis that is institution initiated, the professional is the bearer of the "bad news." For many of us, this means inflicting pain on unsuspecting families, which is something that many in the helping professions tend to shy away from. Our tendency is to immediately mitigate the pain by telling the family something positive, such as "Your child is deaf, but we have cochlear implants that will help your child immensely" or "You are fortunate that we caught this disorder so early." This type of talk is not helpful to families; they can make themselves feel better on their own, and it does not give them sanction to grieve. What they do need at this point is a compassionate listener who will provide information as needed. The professional needs to reframe the bringing of bad news; instead of seeing the delivery of the news as inflicting pain, it should be approached as the beginning of the habilitation process.

Although pain seems to be a necessary component of the diagnostic processes, it is also the initiation of steps to ameliorate the disorder.

Congenital deafness presents a somewhat different diagnostic problem because it is not readily apparent, as is, for example, a cleft palate, and it must be detected through newborn screening, thus necessitating a two-part procedure: the screening and the actual diagnosis. Unfortunately, in most programs the screening is conducted by hospital personnel who have little knowledge of deafness and not necessarily any skill in counseling. The clinical audiologist is often removed from the initial screening, and the first contact between the clinician and parent may occur several weeks later when the hearing loss is confirmed. Parents are left in limbo until the confirmation.

For the parents, there probably could not be a worse time to receive bad news about their newborn than shortly after birth. They have just been through the stress of the birth, hormones are running amok, and they are primed for joy, which is severely dashed. The potential for interfering with parental bonding is high, and confounding the screening procedures is the fact that the false-positive rate for hearing loss in newborns is also elevated. In Massachusetts for the year 2006, the false-positive rate was 75% (Luterman & Kurtzer-White, 1999). The high rate is due in part to the fact that many newborns have a legitimate conductive hearing loss caused by debris in the ear and distortions in the head because of the birth process, but these typically clear up spontaneously in several days.

Although parents of children with confirmed hearing impairment often say that they appreciate finding out so early, when they have a chance to reflect on their experience, they invariably report that they feel cheated at never having had the opportunity to enjoy their newborn in a relaxed way. Almost all parents of children with confirmed hearing impairment agree that the best time to find out about the hearing impairment would be when their child was 3 or 4 months of age (Luterman & Kurtzer-White, 1999). At that point, the parents would have had a chance to enjoy their baby and would be more physically and emotionally receptive to the diagnosis. Testing at 3 or 4 months of age would eliminate most of the false-positives, and I don't think it would significantly delay the habilitation. Also, the parent would be better able to follow through responsibly on professional recommendations. Somehow, professionals need to delay the screening to a later time; this seems to me a logistical problem that is amenable to a solution.

Within the current protocol of screening and notifying within 48 hours of birth, it is absolutely essential that professionals not use the term *failure*. Parents should be told that their child is referred for further testing or that the test has two parts and needs to be completed later. The informing of parents needs to be subtly nuanced so as not to alarm them needlessly but to ensure that they follow through on the recommendation. To this end, hospital personnel who are doing the screening and informing of the parents need ongoing training to ensure that a suitable protocol is followed.

At first blush it may seem very difficult to actively include parents in the test protocols of a newborn. Testing by the audiologist in the confirmation phase is usually done via an auditory brainstem response test and/or an evoked otoacoustic emissions test. Neither of these tests requires the infant to be awake. The tests' results are presented on a moving graph, with a fairly subtle blip indicating a response to the stimulus. At this point, the audiologist can empower the parents by enlisting them as codiagnosticians. The audiologist can sit with the parent and explain the graph; then both, sitting side by side, can watch the graph and decide whether or not there was a response. In this manner, shortly after testing, the decision can be made whether the child responded, and counseling can then proceed as in the parent-driven model.

I cannot emphasize enough the impact that the diagnostic process has on subsequent family–clinician relationships. If we as professionals perform the diagnostic mindfully, with an eye to client empowerment, then subsequent clinicians will reap the benefits of an involved family. If, however, we start the family members off as passive observers of the process and as recipients of our expertise, then the tendency will be to create dependent, passive parents. The diagnostic is a time of imprinting and sets a family–clinician dynamic that is difficult to change in subsequent encounters. My fear is that with institution-driven diagnosis, the tendency is to maintain control, with the professional serving as both the initiator and bearer of the bad news. Only if we are mindful and creative can we create collaborative diagnostic processes with institution-driven diagnosis. It is well worth the effort.

TECHNIQUES OF COUNSELING

I approach writing this chapter with some trepidation. If students concentrate solely on their counseling technique, their effectiveness can be severely limited. Good counseling technique flows from personality; it is seamless. Technique should not be readily apparent to the person being counseled or to an observer. This is not to say that there is no technique or that there is no discipline to be learned by the student. As the counselor gains more experience and becomes more secure, technique is incorporated into personality; the skill then becomes unconscious. I find that I frequently have to invent a reason why I did something when a student observer questions me in postevaluation sessions. Counseling is something I just "do"; if I am conscious of technique, I become mechanical and the technique fails because it interferes with the authenticity of the relationship. If the clients know they are being counseled, the counselor is probably doing it poorly.

Counseling is not a mantle that the professional puts on when a client is present and then discards the rest of the time. It is an attitude, something that is lived. I do not see how one can be a caring, responsive person only within the context of a client–professional relationship, and not in other aspects of one's life. Counseling, as I view it, is an integrated approach to all interpersonal relationships; one "counsels" everybody who approaches in a caring and responsive manner. The techniques employed by a counselor will flow from personality and personal congruence, as well as from a counseling philosophy that has been incorporated into the way in which the counselor approaches clients.

Each counselor develops a personal paradigms framework of thought, which is a personal strategy for understanding and explaining certain aspects of reality, a filter built from an individual's life experiences, prejudices, and constructs. A paradigm is the central organizer of how each person views reality. Events are filtered through our personal paradigms and interpreted by us. In counseling, our paradigms are influenced very heavily by our philosophical notions of how people learn.

In Chapter 2, I discussed four somewhat different ways of viewing the client. The behaviorist sees the client as a mass of conditioned responses; the humanist sees an organism that is seeking to grow; the existentialist sees someone struggling with the great issues of existence (death, freedom/responsibility, loneliness, and meaninglessness); and the cognitivist sees someone who has made unfounded intellectual assumptions about the world that need to be examined. Technique should not be bound to a particular philosophy. Although I like to think of myself as a humanist, I use some techniques that fit well within behavioral or rational-emotive therapy. I think a professional should make therapeutic choices not because of identification with a particular therapy, but rather because the evidence based on clinical experience has tended to indicate that this is the way to be most helpful to the client. Arbuckle (1970) wrote the following passage about this subject:

> In the long run, it would seem that the effective counselor is one who has worked out for himself, through the experience of experimentation, the means by which he can most effectively use himself in the human interaction known as counseling. His orientation has been eclectic, rather than parochial and while his own life is in a constant state of movement and change, he has learned that there are certain modes of operation which are most effective for him, thus there is a degree of consistency in his operation as a counselor. While he is open to consider any means that will work with the client he is aware that his own limitations are such that he cannot be all things for all people. He is acceptant of the thought that there is no model, no method, no technique, which will be consistently successful for him with any other human individual who may come to him as a client. (Arbuckle, 1970, p. 291)

Counselor Control via Response

In a counseling relationship, I wait to hear what issues are on the client's mind before I make a clinical judgment of how best to proceed. There are no stupid questions, only ill-judged responses. The nondirective or person-centered approach affords a great deal of counselor control. The way the counselor elects to respond will to a large extent determine the future course of the counselor–client interaction. The timing of a response is critical: There are times when a client can make good use of content and other times when the content is inappropriate. The counselor needs to select which response would be most facilitative within the context of client interaction. This requires careful listening. If we listen carefully, the client will tell us what is needed.

A father of an autistic child might say, "There are no adequate services for autistic children in this state." I might respond to this statement by doing any one of the following:

- Telling him about the services that are available and offering him a directory of services (content response)

- Asking him how he came to have that opinion (counterquestion)

- Commenting, "That must frighten you when you think about the lack of available services for your child" (affect response)

- Telling him he is correct, and then commenting on what a wonderful opportunity this presents for him to get involved in establishing suitable programs (reframing)

- Telling him about my experience trying to find services for my child (sharing self)

- Responding with a clinical "uh-huh" (affirmation)

None of these responses is necessarily the best one. (I have chosen six possible responses, which seem to me to be the most clinically facilitative.) Each response is appropriate within the context of the relationship. Each response will move the interaction into a different dimension, and the appropriateness is determined by a clinical judgment of the therapeutic context. The clinician must distinguish between the teaching moment and the counseling moment. This is not easy to do when caught up in the relationship interaction. The counseling moments are very often seen in retrospect. The timing of the response is critical, as are many nonverbal features—tone of voice, facial expression, and body language. Let us look at each response in a bit more detail.

Content Response

The content response—the one most commonly used by professionals—generally keeps the relationship at an expected and rather predictable level. In the initial stages of a relationship, the professional provides content to establish credibility; in the latter stages, content is necessary to make appropriate decisions. Generally, content-based relationships are short term. When the professional has a limited amount of time, content predominates and tends to keep waiting rooms clear. A professional has the responsibility to keep current regarding information and to separate fact from opinion—not an easy task. Content has immense value when it is used appropriately but, as I have mentioned several times, content cannot be absorbed when emotions are high.

Counterquestion

I have found that people seldom want advice, even when they seem to be seeking it by asking a question. Through questions, they usually are seeking confirmation of a position or a decision that they have already made. Instead of revealing that decision, they often ask a question in hopes that their decision will be confirmed. Giving advice rarely works: A wise man doesn't need it, and a fool won't take it. I have a sign over my desk that says, "Give me a fish and I eat for a day. Teach me to fish and I eat for the rest of my life." Advice giving is fish giving. People don't learn from it because they take no ownership. If it works they are back for more, and if it fails they curse the giver of the advice, but in either case they have not learned. Often the most protective and facilitative response one can give to a confirmation question is the counterquestion.

The counterquestion forces the person to reveal his or her position. For example, a Spanish-speaking mother of a newly diagnosed deaf son asked me whether she would have to speak English to him at home if she enrolled him in our nursery. I resisted the temptation to tell her that it would be less confusing for her child if she did (she could figure that out for herself) and instead responded by asking her what she wanted to do. The woman responded that if we made her speak English at home, she would not enroll in the nursery. I told her that our policy was to speak English in the nursery and that she could decide what she wanted to do at home. The mother accepted my response and a month later, when she was ready, announced to the parent support group that she was going to speak English at home. At the time of admission to the program, she was not ready to give up her child as both a hearing child and a non-Spanish-speaking child. Parents will usually find the "right" answers for themselves if we give them the time and space to do it. The counterquestion is a very valuable teaching strategy. It forces the learner back onto his or her own resources. The counterquestion response to the client's lament, "You don't answer my questions," is, "Why should I answer your questions?"

Clients' confirmation questions also are used to forestall rejection. A question is a low-risk contribution to an interaction: The questioner does not have to reveal him- or herself; instead, he or she is asking the other person to reveal something. For example, when I am asked if I am busy tonight, I usually respond by asking if the questioner had something in mind for me to do. Embedded in almost all questions is a statement, and I needed to be sensitive enough to respond to the statement or at least to elicit it.

For me, the best indicator of the trust level in a professional–client relationship is the number of question-and-answer interactions. In the initial stages of a relationship, where trust is not high, there are usually a great many questions. As the relationship develops and grows, the client becomes more willing to offer statements and observations. The clinician can facilitate this therapeutic movement by not always answering questions and supplying content. The counterquestion can be a powerful tool for moving the relationship beyond the initial stages.

Affect Response

On the surface, the affect response appears risky, but actually it is a reaction to what Carl Rogers in a lecture called "the faint knocking." By listening very carefully and trying to see the world as the client sees it and reflecting the client's feelings back, the counselor can help to open up the relationship—sometimes very dramatically. The appropriate affect response greatly increases the intimacy level in a relationship. I have found that even an inaccurate response is not harmful; it generally forces people to further clarify their feelings, and in the process of clarification, we both can generally understand the feelings better.

The affect response is very potent in building a counseling relationship. Caring is conveyed by our willingness to listen and be responsive to what the person means and also to what the person cannot quite bring him- or herself to say. Rogers (1951) called this *empathetic listening,* which at first glance would appear to be a readily teachable technique. Unfortunately, empathetic listening is often abused and can come across as parroting and mechanical in the hands of someone who has learned the form but not the substance of the humanistic approach. In an article written for physicians, Sabbeth and Leventhal (1988) talked about the "trial balloons" that patients and families send up when they interact with their doctor, asserting that it is the physician's responsibility to respond to the feelings embedded in those "balloons." I remember one family that I worked with. The husband had recently had a severe stroke, and the wife said almost as an aside, "I can't seem to leave the house anymore without going back to check whether I have locked the door and shut off the stove. Sometimes I go back two or three times." My response to her was, "It seems like you don't trust yourself." This led to a very fruitful discussion about her anxiety and feelings of inadequacy in her ability to cope with her husband's disabilities.

Because the affect response requires considerable follow-up, it is rarely a response that one gives when there is limited time. I find that responding at the affect level is usually more helpful in the initial stages of contact and diagnosis. It allows for a ventilation of emotions and the alleviation of some of the secondary feelings that accompany the strong affect surrounding a catastrophic illness. The wife, for example, who feels angry at her husband for having a stroke can be given the opportunity to talk about her feelings of anger without feeling guilty. In later stages, when affect is not predominant, I generally give more content responses or reframe experiences into something more positive.

Reframing

The timing of reframing has to be precise and it cannot be used too frequently, or the professional will be accused of being a Pollyanna. The technique is immensely effective in mobilizing the person to look at the positive side. Good reframing always gives the person a jolt. It should cause the person to stop short and examine the assumptions underlying his or her statement. We as professionals can be so focused on a problem that we seldom see the challenge that is present in the situation. Reframing encourages responsibility assumption. The parent who complains about the "dumb questions" he gets from strangers who see his child's hearing aids can be brought up short by the response, "What a marvelous opportunity to educate someone about deafness."

Professionals can also benefit from the reframing response by looking for the positive when analyzing their client relationships. For example, the same behavior can be interpreted as stubborn or as determined. If the clinician is always looking at the client's stubborn side, he or she will have a negative view of the client. A determined client has a much greater chance of success than a stubborn one.

I think that we seldom consider or call attention to a client's strengths, because we are so often looking at the deficits. It helps, when I supervise student clinicians, to ask them, "What does this child have going for him?" and then, "How can we capitalize on those strengths?" When we focus on the client's strengths, somehow the problem begins to disappear far faster than when we emphasize the deficits. It might seem that there are limits to situations that can be reframed but that might not be so. I remember watching a video of Kubler-Ross counseling a woman in the terminal stages of amyotrophic lateral sclerosis (ALS). The woman was totally paralyzed and being cared for by her two daughters. Through one of her daughters, who bent close to her barely moving lips, she asked Kubler-Ross, "What good am I?" and Kubler-Ross's response, without batting an eye, was, "You are giving your daughters a chance to pay you back for all the care you gave them," which seemed to satisfy the woman.

I have several favorite ways of reframing in response to the question, "Why me?" I might respond, "Why not you?" To families with children newly diagnosed as disabled, I might say, "This child has guaranteed you an interesting life." I try to reframe all "mistakes" into "nuggets of gold" whereby the person learned something valuable. I might comment to a client that his disability is a powerful teacher for him (and can be for others as well). I have personally found this notion of "teacher" in disability very potent. This notion also works with interpersonal and clinical relationships. I can reframe difficult clients into potent teachers for me, and I can do the same with previously obnoxious colleagues and acquaintances. If I approach them as people who have something to give me so that I grow, then the quality of the interaction changes markedly. For the astute businessperson, the complaining customer is a best friend, because that customer is helping improve the product. With such an attitude, you can change the world.

Reframing as a technique and as a life tool is very powerful. For all of the possible responses, but especially reframing, timing is critical. It is very easy to lose people by reframing too early in the grief process; an ill-timed or ill-delivered reframing response can be seen as offensive. On the other hand, the ultimate goal of counseling is to help the clients reframe their life situations into something positive. When this is done by the clients themselves, the counselor's job is finished because there is no longer any problem.

Sharing Self

The image of the "professional" that most of us have is of someone who is in total control at all times. This is someone who knows the answers and, therefore, is someone the client looks up to. In practice, we know that this is not true, that there are times when we (the "professionals") are out of control in our personal and professional lives. Standard clinical practice says we should hide this from our clients. I have found, however, that it is sometimes very helpful and facilitative to share our own doubts and uncertainties with clients. If we always seem in control, clients tend to feel very inadequate. A father of a child with Down syndrome said, "I like to see the teacher have a hard time with my son. It validates my experience, too." Sometimes the most helpful thing we can say to a parent might be, "I haven't the foggiest idea what to do right now with your child. Do you have any ideas?" This empowers the parent and humanizes us at the same time. (I wouldn't suggest using this response early in the relationship; it should be saved until a great deal of trust has been established.)

Sharing self also means sharing our feelings by being willing to tell clients that we are angry at them. This is an opportunity to work out issues in the relationship. Few professionals let themselves get angry with clients directly. More often they ventilate on colleagues or repress the anger, which usually subverts the therapy. Similarly, professionals don't always share positive feelings with their clients. Sharing self reveals our authenticity as fellow human beings. A fear that most beginning clinicians seem to have is about crying with the client when painful material is revealed. I see crying with the client as a sharing-self response, which almost invariably will bring client and clinician closer. The clinician will be revealed as caring and compassionate, which can only work to deepen the relationship.

It is valuable to the client to realize that the professional is also a person who has concerns, fears, and a life outside of the clinic. This revelation helps the client assume responsibility and prevents the professional from being elevated to the guru category. The timing of using this response is especially critical. If it is done too early, the professional will lose credibility at a time when credibility establishment is critical for the relationship. The sharing-self responses should usually emerge later in the relationship and with clients who have a relatively high degree of self-esteem.

Affirmation

When I think of affirmation, I am reminded of the countless cartoons featuring a psychoanalyst: A patient is on the couch talking, and the psychiatrist is asleep; presumably progress is being made. Very often the client just needs a sounding board; he or she needs permission to talk and to express feelings without judgment. Affirmation responses can be statements such as "That must be very hard" or "That's okay" or "Uh-huh." When in doubt, it is best to affirm; it can be used in almost all situations. The "uh-huh" response with appropriate nonverbal behavior can be very helpful in unleashing the client's feelings. The "uh-huh" is also an affirmation that the counselor has heard the client, and an invitation for the client to continue. I have a poster in my office given to me by a group of students that says, "It often shows a fine command of language to say nothing." Sometimes the most facilitative remarks are the ones that you do not deliver.

Deciding How to Respond

The clinician has a wide array of potential responses; which one is selected can determine the direction of the relationship with the client. There are no "right" responses, only different roads to travel. If the response you give moves the relationship in a fruitful direction, then it is appropriate. It is also quite possible to recover from taking a less fruitful route. I have found that if something is important, it keeps coming up, and a feeling is seldom lost; it gets reworked and emerges again. Again I emphasize that the nonverbal elements in interactions are also important, perhaps more important than what is actually said.

The following selected questions and statements were made by clients or family members. The reader may want to use them to practice the various responses discussed in this chapter. Below each statement are some possible responses. These are only some of the multiple possibilities of responding. As I've said, there are no right or wrong answers, but different responses will move the clinical interaction in different directions; it is the context that will determine the value of the response. Clinicians are constantly making choices even if they are not aware of them at the time. The art of counseling is in reading the context and selecting the most facilitative response. I am not sure this skill can be taught but only learned through experience.

1. "If this were your child (parent), what would you do?"

    Comment: This frequently asked question, which reflects the speaker's insecurity and feelings of being overwhelmed, could be reflected back as "It sounds like you are feeling insecure right now." Ultimately this discussion will lead to contracting, and roles and responsibilities can be delineated. Answering with content will tend to create and support dependency in the parent.

2. "Are cochlear implants any good?"

    Comment: This question, which is clearly seeking confirmation, is best answered with a counterquestion: "What have you heard about implants?"

3. "My husband's family is very unemotional."

    Comment: An affect response, such as "That must leave you feeling very alone," can be effective. An affirmation response, such as "That must be so hard," can also be very facilitative.

4. "Will I have to be present when you test my husband?"

    Comment: If you have time, this type of affect response might be most helpful: "It must be so hard for you to sit there and see him fail." With limited time, you might go for confirmation by asking, "Would you like to be present?"

5. "Is it true that graduates of schools for the deaf are only able to read on a third-grade level?"

    Comment: A useful affect response might be, "That must be pretty frightening for you." Also, confirmation may be sought: "Where did you get that statistic?"

6. "What causes stuttering (any disability) in a child?"

   Comment: This is a red-flag comment indicating very dangerous waters. Usually, parents have a suspicion about what they might have done to cause the child's disability. This is the "guilty secret," and this simple query can become the key to unlocking the door. If you respond with content, you may inadvertently confirm a parent's worse fears. Best to go for confirmation by asking, "Do you think you did something to cause your child to stutter?"

7. "Will my baby (spouse) ever learn to speak?"

   Comment: A query such as this usually reflects insecurity about whether the speaker is doing the right thing to achieve a goal. I frequently respond by saying, "I can't predict the future, but this is a marvelous goal and let's both work hard to accomplish it." I do not reassure but I might affirm by saying, "It must be so hard for you to live with this uncertainty."

8. "My husband comes home and just plays with her."

   Comment: You can respond with affect—for example, "It sounds like you are angry at him for not sharing the responsibility"—or you can reframe—for example, "It's great that somebody in the family is playing with her."

9. "My wife can't stand the sound of the artificial larynx."

   Comment: You can respond with affect by saying, for example, "That must be very scary for you" or "It seems like your voice is affecting your marriage," or you can affirm by commenting, "That must be so hard for you."

10. "You don't answer any of my questions."

    Comment: This is an invitation to work out the roles in the relationship by responding, "It seems like you want me to tell you what to do," or to respond to the affect by replying, "This must be very irritating for you." The latter response might inflame the speaker further.

Case Studies: Hypothetical Families

The hypothetical families presented here are fictionalized case studies designed to illuminate particular problems. I have used these case studies in classes I teach to speech pathology majors, for in-service workshops, and, less frequently, in parent groups. I found them very useful for me in my early work with groups when I needed the comfort of more structure and direction in my role as the leader. I seldom use them now because I prefer a much less structured experience.

The first 10 of the following case studies have been adapted from a *Volta Review* article (Luterman, 1969). These cases all involved deafness, but the problems illuminated by the case studies are universal. Interested readers may use the cases as is or may alter them to reflect any other disability or to suit the needs of a particular group.

Case Study 1

Mrs. A. is very confused. She has taken her 2½-year-old son, who is neither talking nor seeming to respond to sound, to several physicians. Her pediatrician has told her that he thought her child was deaf but that nothing could be done until he was 4 years old. One physician has told her that he thinks the child has mental retardation. Her husband and her in-laws, on the other hand, feel that there is nothing wrong with the child, and that he will "outgrow it." They tell her about an uncle who did not begin talking until he was 4 years of age and who is now perfectly normal. What should Mrs. A. do?

Case Study 2

Mrs. B. sometimes says to herself, "Why did this happen to me?" She has said, "I know I shouldn't feel this way, but I really resent having a deaf child. He takes so much of my energy and time. He is so difficult for me to control; I worry about him so much. Every now and then, I find myself wishing for a moment that I had never had him, and then I feel guilty about feeling that way. I also hate to go out with him because of his screaming and because of the stares of passersby when they see his hearing aid. I just can't stand strangers' questions and well-meaning advice any longer." What can be done about Mrs. B.'s feelings?

Case Study 3

Mrs. C. feels that her deaf child was given to her because of her past "sins." She has devoted herself to taking care of her child; she no longer goes out socially and has dropped most of her friends. She spends a good part of the day working with the deaf child and taking him to his therapy lessons; she spends evenings reading and talking about deafness. She does not trust any babysitters. Mr. C. has begun to complain about feeling neglected, and he says he is concerned about the two older children, who have not received much attention from their mother. What are your feelings about the C. family?

Case Study 4

Dr. D. is a physician whose father and grandfather were also doctors. He has always wanted to have a son who would be a physician, too. Since he has learned that his only child is deaf and therefore will never be able to be a physician, Dr. D. has not devoted much attention to the boy. He has said, "I had so many plans for him. Every time I see the hearing aid, it reminds me that he won't be what I would like him to be, and it's really very hard for me to be with him. I know I shouldn't feel that way and it probably is harmful to him, but having a deaf son is a very big disappointment to me." What can that father do?

Case Study 5

Mr. and Mrs. E. have three children. Their youngest is a 2-year-old deaf child; the other two are 6 and 10 years of age. The parents have been very busy taking the 2-year-old to various clinics for evaluations, and they have begun a twice-weekly therapy program and lessons at home. The middle child has responded to his younger brother's problem very well and, in fact, seems more understanding of it than the oldest boy. The oldest child has reacted with a great deal of jealousy. He is extremely difficult to manage; he throws violent tantrums and often simply withdraws for fairly long periods of time. Mr. E. has reacted to that behavior with stiff disciplinary measures. Mrs. E.'s reactions have varied from anger to pleading and bribing. At the same time, she recognizes that neither she nor her husband is handling the 10-year-old effectively. What might they do?

Case Study 6

Mr. and Mrs. F. have a 2-year-old deaf son. Mrs. F.'s parents live very near them, and Mrs. Z. has not accepted the fact that her grandson is deaf and will "never" be able to hear. She keeps sending her daughter articles from newspapers and magazines about operations and cures for deafness. She is constantly urging her daughter to take him to one more doctor. Mrs. F. says, "It is hard enough for us to accept our child's deafness, but it is especially difficult when we keep having to explain it over and over again to other people who don't really listen to us."

Mr. F.'s parents, on the other hand, live farther away and see their grandchild rather infrequently. When they do see their grandson, they feel he should not be punished—"After all, he is deaf." They become upset if either Mr. or Mrs. F. disciplines the deaf child in their presence. How can that family be helped to reduce some of these conflicts?

Case Study 7

Timothy G. is a 3½-year-old deaf child with no siblings. He is not permitted outside the house unless accompanied by one of his parents, despite the fact that he lives on a quiet suburban street. His mother is very concerned that he might be hit by a child on a bicycle or by a car because he cannot hear. The parents are also afraid that he might fall down and hurt his ear with the hearing aid. Consequently, he seldom leaves his home or plays with children his own age. Should that situation be altered? Why? Why not? If so, what suggestions would you make to the parents?

Case Study 8

Mr. and Mrs. H. live in a medium-sized town, 40 miles from Boston. They have lived in the town all their lives; Mr. H. owns and operates a small business there. They own their home in the community, and both are very active in community affairs. They have three children, ages 10, 8, and 5, the youngest of whom is deaf and has been accepted in a school for the deaf in a suburb near Boston. Because of the distance involved, the school will accept the child only on a residential basis. Rather than have her daughter board at the school, Mrs. H. wants to move to a community close to the school so that her daughter can attend on a daily basis. Mr. H. is opposed to such a move; he feels that moving to the new community would disrupt the whole family. What should that family do?

Case Study 9

Mr. and Mrs. I. find themselves at complete odds over the management of their deaf 3-year-old son. Mrs. I. is convinced of the worth of the aural–oral approach and is trying to teach her son to lip-read and communicate orally. Mr. I., on the other hand, is convinced that only a very small percentage of deaf persons ever attain reasonable oral communication skills. He would prefer that his son learn manual communication, so he can at least communicate easily with other deaf persons. Mr. I. is around his children very seldom, but whenever he is, he uses manual signs to communicate with his deaf son. What can these parents do?

Case Study 10

Mr. and Mrs. J. have a 3-year-old deaf child. The family lives on an island and, because of the lack of facilities and professional help, Mrs. J. has had the sole responsibility for teaching her daughter. The child is doing well; she lip-reads about 30 words at this time, responds very well to contextual cues, and can use about 15 words expressively. Mrs. J. has placed her child in a nursery school with hearing children, where she also does well; the mother has just been told that her daughter can begin attending a school for the deaf on the mainland, which means that the child can get home only every 4 to 6 weeks. What should she do?

Case Study 11

Mr. and Mrs. K. have recently divorced. Mrs. K. has retained custody of their 3-year-old autistic son. The court has given Mr. K. permission to visit the child once a week. Mrs. K. finds that her ex-husband's visits are very unsettling to both her and their son. She feels that the child cannot understand why his father leaves and is not home during the week; the child is very confused by the whole situation. Mr. K. also brings a great many presents when he comes, and takes the child to exciting places; by contrast, Mrs. K. feels that she looks very "bad" to the child and she is upset at the unfairness of the arrangement. What can this family do to relieve some of the tensions?

Case Study 12

Mr. and Mrs. L. recently attended an Individualized Education Program (IEP) meeting at which the presiding educators unanimously voiced the opinion that their 3-year-old child should go to the local school for the deaf. However, that school only offers a program in total communication. The child has been attending an aural–oral nursery school and has been doing quite well in developing her speech and language skills. The parents want her to continue in the aural mode and would like their child to attend a hearing nursery and receive tutorial help. They feel that the educators are suggesting the school for the deaf because it is expedient and not because it is the best facility for their child. The first IEP meeting ended in a deadlock, and all parties agreed to meet again in 2 weeks. What strategies should the parents employ for the next meeting?

Case Study 13

Mr. and Mrs. M. have recently found out that their 2-year-old child is deaf. They have one other, older child who hears normally. Mrs. M. has a deaf brother and a deaf uncle; consequently, she feels somehow responsible for the child's deafness. Mr. M. has not been helpful. He also blames Mrs. M. for causing the child's deafness and has left all the responsibility for the child's education to her. On one level, Mrs. M. deeply resents having that responsibility; on another level, she accepts it as her "punishment." What can Mrs. M. do to alter the unhealthy home situation?

Case Study 14

Mr. and Mrs. N.'s 11-year-old child has cerebral palsy and is deeply resentful of being disabled. He is constantly questioning Mr. N. about why he is disabled and refuses to believe that he will not outgrow it. He is currently being mainstreamed and is doing quite well academically; however, he has few friends among his classmates and he does not want to have anything to do with other people with disabilities. What can Mr. and Mrs. N. do to help their son?

Case Study 15

Mr. and Mrs. O. are a couple in their 30s who have recently adopted an 18-month-old child, only to discover that the child is multiply handicapped. The adoption is not yet official, and the parents have the choice of returning the child to the agency and going on the waiting list for another child. Mrs. O. wants to keep the child because she has grown attached to him and feels that she can be a good parent of a child with disabilities. Mr. O. believes that they should return the child to the agency before they get any more attached. He feels that being a parent is hard enough and that being the parent of a child with disabilities is asking for too much trouble. He is not sure he has the resources to be a good parent to that child, and Mrs. O. feels she cannot raise the child without the full support of her husband. What can that family do?

Locus of Control

Central to all counseling techniques is the notion of locus of control. Rotter (1966), a social psychologist, developed a scale that measures whether an individual has an internal or external locus of control. According to Rotter, people with an internal locus of control tend to feel that they have personal power and can control their own destiny, whereas people with an external locus of control feel that they are controlled by others. "Externals" believe that things just happen to them as the result of luck or fate. "Internals" feel their lives are "them doing them." Locus of control is conceived as a continuum, with most people located between the extremes of total control (inner locus) and total powerlessness (external locus). Counseling technique, I believe, has to cede control to the client so that ultimately the client feels responsible and powerful. In short, counseling seeks to empower clients by moving the locus of control in an inward direction.

Because behaviorists view clients as a mass of conditioned responses controlled by others, behavioral counseling techniques, if used too extensively and inappropriately, tend to encourage clients to have an external locus of control. A careful behavioral counselor teaches the client to identify the reinforcers in the environment and then teaches counterconditioning techniques. Clients in the hands of a competent behavioral therapist can develop an inner locus of control.

Within the sphere of humanistic counseling, control is always vested in the clients. Therefore, it is easier for them to develop an inner locus of control because they have been given responsibility over their learning from the inception of therapy.

The concept of locus of control has received some research attention in communication disorders. Although the studies cited here appear dated, they are still very much relevant to current populations. There are no contradictory studies. Dowaliby, Burke, and McKee (1983) modified the Rotter (1966) scale for use with deaf subjects and found that students with hearing impairment entering college were substantially more external in their locus of control than a control sample of students with normal hearing. White (1982) reported on a series of workshops he conducted with 281 teachers and counselors at six schools for the deaf. The participants were asked to rank 24 social competencies on the basis of what deaf children need to accomplish most. Almost all participants rated "accepting responsibilities for own actions" as the most important issue for deaf students. Bodner and Johns (1977) used the Rotter scale with 38 deaf students and found that they were significantly more external in their locus of control than the subjects with normal hearing.

The failure to take responsibility for one's actions in the adult deaf population was recently and vividly brought home to me. I lectured at a conference attended by a large number of deaf adults, and my speech was interpreted. After the speech, which was an hour long, a deaf adult who was sitting in the back of the room complained vigorously that he missed the entire speech because he could not see the interpreter. The conference organizer, to whom I spoke afterward, felt guilty about the incident until we talked about it. She then realized that the responsibility was not hers. The deaf man could have moved his seat or complained at the onset of the lecture, and the interpreter would have moved. Instead, he made a choice to sit there and then complain about it later when nothing could be done about it.

Locus of control has also been studied in stuttering populations. Craig, Franklin, and Andrews (1985) used the specially constructed Locus of Control of Behavior Scale on 17 stutterers in therapy. The researchers found that clients who moved toward internality in locus of control were more likely to maintain improvement over time. Relapse was more likely for those who did not internalize. Madison, Budd, and Itzkowitz (1986) found that stuttering children who showed greater internality also showed greater improvement following treatment than those children with a relatively external locus of control.

Locus of control has not been adequately researched in training programs. Only one study stands out. Shirlberg et al. (1977) examined locus of control in communication disorder majors. They found that students who have an internal locus of control were rated as better clinicians than those with an external locus of control. As the authors so aptly wrote, "Excellent clinicians do in fact view themselves as pilots rather than pawns of their fate" (p. 315).

Populations with disabilities have also been studied in regard to locus of control and, as one might expect, they have generally been found to have an external locus of control. Hallahan, Gasar, Cohen, and Tarver (1978) found that 28 matched teenagers with learning disabilities were significantly more external in their locus of control orientation than were control subjects. Land and Vineberg (1965) reported that blind subjects were more externally oriented then their sighted controls.

The finding of external locus of control in populations with disabilities is not surprising when one considers how professionals tend to interact with them. It is not uncommon to see professionals who are constantly "rescuing" clients; they don't want clients to experience additional failure or pain. In doing this, however, a clinician promotes an external locus of control that makes populations with disabilities—already dependent for so many things—feel that others are more powerful and more capable than they are.

Encouraging a more internal locus of control in our client populations is as much a matter of attitude as it is of clinical technique. The attitude we must convey to clients is that they are capable and that they have control of many aspects of their lives. The notion that the client always has control of how he or she will react to the disability is paramount. (Although a person may have no choice about being disabled, he or she always has a choice about what to do about the disability.) The clinical techniques employed in helping clients should generally be covert and not obvious to clients or to observers. Many times we can be most helpful by not doing anything except being there as responsive, caring human beings, allowing the clients to work things out for themselves. Sometimes the very effective clinician creates vacuums that the clients have to fill, thus forcing clients to act and to take responsibility for their actions; in so doing, there is growth. Lesson plans, for example, need to be mutually arrived at, with the client participating fully in planning the course of therapy. Asking children what toys they would like to play with or, as mentioned previously, when completing diagnostics, asking the clients what they need to know invests some control in them. In group meetings (discussed in the next chapter), I never call on participants; they are allowed to sit quietly as long as they like. The clinical silence or vacuum becomes a powerful teaching tool that, unfortunately, is not always appreciated by supervisors.

Language Changing

Language changing is a cognitive technique based on the rational-emotive therapy developed by Ellis (1977), which is more fully described in Chapter 2. Language changing derives from the clinical applications of general semantics. In this technique, the professional pays careful attention to the client's language, which illuminates the underlying and sometimes irrational assumptions the client is making. I have a poster in my office that says, "The shape of my world is the shape of my language." During an interaction I sometimes gently point out to the client the assumption underlying the words he or she is using. For example, the use of "have to" almost always reflects an external locus of control. When a parent said to me, "I have to try acupuncture," I said, "Don't you mean 'choose to'?" and a bit later, "Why do you feel you have to?" This was an invitation for the parent to look at the feeling of being driven and controlled by others. In this particular case, her own guilt was driving her. "But" always reflects an underlying ambivalence. I might respond to a statement such as, "I want to speak in public but I am afraid," with the response, "Can't you be afraid and still speak in public?" This encourages acting in the face of fear; the "but" allows wallowing in ambivalence. I always examine carefully all the "Yes . . . but . . ." statements, which reflect ambivalence. "Should" and "ought" reflect guilt, deficiency, and a sense of failing. Constructs such as, "I should talk to my pediatrician about his misdiagnosis of my child's hearing," might receive a response such as, "Do you want to talk to your physician?" "Should" and "ought" are also very reflective of an external locus of control, and changing them to "choose to" or "choose not to" encourages a more internal locus and assumption of responsibility for behavior.

We need to help clients recognize the choices they are making. I always examine the clients' language to see where they are evading responsibility. Evasion happens frequently when clients use the pronoun "we" instead of "I," as in, "We are unhappy with this class." I might respond, "Do you mean *you* are unhappy?" One indicator of a shift in locus of control is the spontaneous use of the "I" form, which reflects ownership of behavior. When clients make that shift, I know that we are well on our way to a successful counseling interaction.

When someone says she has been "lucky," I might change the word to "good." If a client says, "I was lucky to have him for a husband," I might respond, "You were good, so therefore he married you." It is very helpful to take credit for the good we do; most "lucky" people take all the responsibility for the bad and very little credit for the good. This is a hard way to live.

I don't allow clients to use collective nouns, such as "men" and "women." When I hear a sentence such as, "All men are lousy," I change it to, "The men in your life have been lousy," and then I might gently comment, "It sounds as if you have not been meeting the right men." (I also might comment, "You sound pretty angry.")

Linguistic changes need to be made gently. The timing is critical. I seldom make linguistic changes during the initial stages of diagnosis or when affect is high because changing language forces the client into a cognitive stance. The client's trust in the professional also needs to be high, or the linguistic alterations can be seen as interfering and annoying.

Silence

Silence is an important component of any therapeutic relationship. A long, embarrassed silence frequently occurs early in my clinical interactions. Because clients generally expect me, the professional, to direct conversation, when I do not take the lead, a silence ensues. It is vital that I do not break this silence. It tells the clients that if they want something to happen in this relationship, they have to act. The silence is a primary vehicle for responsibility assumption, and it is vital that I do not take that responsibility from the clients. Discomfort with silence initially forces many young clinicians to act; they then become role bound to make things happen while the clients sit back and watch.

Silences are generally uncomfortable in conventional relationships. I can remember the long painful silences I had as an adolescent on a blind date while I thought frantically of something to say. (I suspect the girl was similarly occupied, but I was too concerned with my own discomfort to think of hers.) The discomfort generated by the clinical silence can be used to motivate action by the clients. Because I am fortified by the knowledge of what I am doing and the value of this technique, I can outwait most clients. The general reaction to the silence is anger; if this surfaces, it becomes a useful vehicle for discussing role expectations.

Later in relationships, the silences that occur are more reflective in nature and are quite comfortable. As intimacy develops, the silences become a valuable learning time for processing material. Where there is silence, there is usually growth. Cook (1964) analyzed the amount of silence in taped therapy sessions and found that the more successful sessions had more silence than those judged to be less successful. Sometimes talking can be used as a smokescreen to hide feelings, but silence often forces one to confront oneself and to experience feelings. A student in a support group commented, "I now realize that the learning is in the silence." (She got an "A.")

Four kinds of silences occur in the counseling relationship. It is critical for the counselor to be able to recognize the kind and quality of each silence.

The Embarrassed Silence

The embarrassed silence usually occurs early in the interaction; the client (or group) is expecting the counselor to act and fill the void, and the counselor doesn't do as expected. It is critical that the counselor not break the silence. This is the empowering silence: The discomfort generated by this silence in the client becomes a powerful motivator for client action. It is a mobilizing force. A parent in a group once said to me,

> I get the feeling sometimes as though there is a big lump of time out there on the table and when it gets silent, it just fritters away and I get very anxious. At times I get angry at you for not speaking and telling me things. I realize now that if I want something to happen here, I have to act, and that is a good thing for me.

Embarrassed silences diminish almost to nonexistence over the life span of the relationship. In a well-functioning group, participants come to relish the silence as a time for reflection.

Changing-Topic Silence

The changing-topic silence occurs in groups and in one-on-one counseling while the individuals reflect on whether they have more to say on the topic at hand. The counselor can use the silence to introduce a topic of concern, although it is best to do that after enough silences have occurred that the group or individual realizes that the counselor is not taking the responsibility for filling the silence. Generally I find that if I have a topic of concern, I bring this up at the meeting's outset. This clears my head so I am able to listen rather than wait for a chance to introduce my topic.

The Reflective Silence

The reflective silence invariably follows some emotionally laden material. This silence is a time-out to think about and to experience the feelings that have been brought to the surface. The reflective silence—a very heavy, palpable feeling in the relationship—takes a great effort to break. I think the deepest feelings take place in silence, and I think all of the really important work is done in silence. I like the Gian Vincenzo Gravina quote, "A bore is someone who deprives you of solitude without providing you with company." I always relish the companionship of a thoughtful silence. Group meetings very often end on this silence, and the feelings generated by it are discussed on another day.

The Termination Silence

Sometimes a client or group lapses into a silence toward the end of a session that has the quality of the changing-topic silence, except that the group or individual is tired and the work for that day is done. Occasionally, I have misinterpreted the termination silence and thought it was the pause before a new topic was to be introduced. I have learned now to check with groups on these occasions to determine if they are finished.

Contracting

In contracting—a technique used extensively in the behavioral approach to counseling—the assumptions underlying the clinician–client relationship are made explicit. The client is required to be explicit about what he or she wants from the clinician, and the clinician is explicit about what he or she will or will not do for the client. Initial sessions are devoted almost solely to the contracting issue. Periodically, as the relationship progresses, time is taken to renegotiate the contract if needed.

I find it very important to delineate carefully what I expect from clients. Many relationships fail because of expectations that are implicit and not complementary. Clients, for example, who expect the therapist to rescue them and a therapist who expects the clients to be very proactive, will have a difficult time unless they can negotiate the differences. If the issue of expectations is not dealt with, the relationship will deteriorate and anger will develop, although it probably will be deflected at an inappropriate source.

Basically, a contract specifies how long the relationship will last, what it will entail, and what the purpose is. Contracts do not have to be detailed or legalistic, but they have to be understood by everybody. In particular, I think the time issue needs to be very clear. Before I start a session, I am always explicit about how much time I have in a given encounter, and I am very rigid about terminating when I said I would. I very seldom extend a session beyond the contracted time. The limited time then serves as an impetus (death awareness) to the clients to work toward solving their problems. If I had an open-ended commitment, clients would tend to avoid dealing with painful material, thinking that they could get to it at some vague future date. It is no accident that more affect-laden material is revealed at the session's end than at the beginning.

I remain open to renegotiating contracts. As relationships change, needs change. I never unilaterally change a relationship; the change has to be discussed and agreed upon. Sometimes the client and I cannot arrive at a mutually satisfactory contract. When this happens, we terminate. I generally refer the client, if he or she initiates the request, to someone who I think can meet the client's needs. I usually give more than one option so the client has a choice. I have ceased trying to be all things to all people, and I recognize that there are some people I cannot help or, more accurately, choose not to help, because to do so would violate my personal values. Invariably, the irresolvable issue is responsibility assumption, where the client persistently wants me to assume much more responsibility than I think is prudent for effecting growth.

Counselor Feedback

The counselor's feelings about a client should be judiciously shared with the client. Although this sharing can facilitate client growth, it must always be done within a context of support, and the timing must be precise. For example, one participant in a student clinician group was especially verbose and continually repeated herself. Toward the end of one of her monologues, I interrupted and commented, "Anne, I find your initial statements and thoughts very interesting, but when you keep repeating yourself, I find myself getting bored and emotionally distanced from you." The comment encouraged her to begin talking about how other people had given her similar feedback and that her verbosity reflected her loneliness and insecurity. The rest of the group, which up to that point had been sitting with glazed-over eyes, began to give her more feedback, which proceeded into a fruitful discussion of loneliness and the things people sometimes do that distance other people.

When feedback is given, it is very important that the person who delivers the feedback take ownership of his or her feelings. Thus, I did not say, "You talk too much," which would have put her on the defensive; I spoke only about what was going on in my mind. As presented, the problem was mine, not hers; as long as I talk about myself, I am always an expert.

Effectiveness of Counseling

A frequent mistake made by the neophyte counselor is in thinking that the goal of counseling is to eliminate the client's pain. This idea is very natural in helping professionals; however, it is not fruitful to take responsibility for another's pain by trying to make the person feel better. It is seldom useful to say or imply that a person should not feel pain; it invalidates the feeling. This strategy generally causes people to feel guilty about their emotional pain. When people we care about are in pain, often it feels like we have failed, and if they can sense our discomfort they often become reluctant to share their feelings with us.

It is not a good thing to express our painful feelings because it imposes pain on others. My grandson, when he was 4 years old, was left in my care for several days. On the first day we went to a playground, a zoo, and lunch at a fast-food restaurant. At home we watched *Lion King* and played Candy Land. After his bedtime story, an exhausted grandfather and exhausted grandson were ready for bed and he said, "I miss my mommy and daddy." Threatened grandfather then responded with, "Look at all the nice things we did today" (my grandson knew all of that), which also said to him that he had no right to feel the way he did and that the honest expressions of his feelings are painful to me. Unfortunately because of grandfather ineptitude, my grandson learned that it was not safe to share his painful feelings. A much more facilitative response would have been,

"You must love them very much" or "That must make you sad," but I did not find it at the time—only after I had reflected about it.

Emotional pain is normal. I expect people to feel sad when bad things happen to them; if I do not encounter pain in people who have a communication disorder or a family member with one, I wonder how they are dealing with this catastrophe. A mother of a newly diagnosed deaf child told me that she was "doing this badly" because she was crying for several hours every day. I assured her that she was not doing badly, but was reacting normally. We as professionals can be most helpful to clients by eliminating the negative feelings about the pain they are experiencing; however, we cannot take away the pain. A core level of pain will remain in those dealing with any permanent disability. The goal of counseling is to detach the feelings from self-defeating behavior. I try to never judge feelings; they simply exist and I accept them. I can, however, work with clients on what constitutes constructive behavior. Thus, a parent who says, "I can feel guilty and I can still act in a way that is in my own and my child's best interests," has grown successfully. Clients find, over time and with careful professional attention, that feelings no longer control them, and "guilty" parents do not have to overprotect their children. Client behavior has to be the ultimate criterion by which we judge the effectiveness of counseling. With time and help, the feelings transform into productive behavior. The anger becomes the energy to make changes; the guilt becomes commitment. The confusion is the spur to learning, and the vulnerability becomes the impetus to reshuffle values. The pain transforms into compassion, especially for all families grappling with a disability.

Professional Humility

If one is to counsel from a humanistic frame of reference—to accept and not prescribe—then one must learn professional humility. Fortunately for me, a marvelous "nugget of gold" occurred rather early in my counseling career. My first clinical experiences stayed with me as though imprinting in my professional infancy. I can still, nearly 30 years later, recall this family very vividly.

Johnny was a 2-year-old hearing-impaired child in the nursery group. He would enter the nursery with his thumb in his mouth and his little finger stuck up one nostril. The finger stayed in his mouth the whole 2 hours of the nursery day, which included 30 minutes of individual speech-language therapy. It was rather hard to relate to someone with his thumb in his mouth and almost impossible for the child to speak. Johnny never participated in nursery activities, preferring to watch the other children. The staff became convinced that he was emotionally disturbed. One goal of therapy was to condition Johnny to remove his thumb from his mouth; another goal was to get Johnny's parents to seek professional counseling help. I assumed the latter responsibility, sitting next to his mother during nursery activities and during speech therapy and pointing out to her how deficient Johnny was compared with the other children.

The mother refused to see any of his nonparticipatory behavior as abnormal. She always seemed to have an explanation for his behavior. Consequently, the clinic was unsuccessful on both counts: The thumb remained in the child's mouth until the end of the semester, and the parents decided, much to our dismay and over our objections, to put Johnny in a hearing nursery school and provide him with individual speech and language therapy. So, with much staff head shaking, the parents left the program. Several months later, I chanced to meet the father socially and of course wanted to know how Johnny was doing. He told me with a big smile on his face, "Johnny kissed his teacher." Well, I thought, at least they got his hand out of his mouth—or did they? The family moved to the West Coast and, as often happens, we lost all contact.

Several years later I happened to be at a meeting on the West Coast and met Johnny's mother. (She had decided to become a speech pathologist.) She came armed to our meeting with all his school records, and I found out that Johnny was attending his neighborhood school, fully mainstreamed, and—as shown by his recent achievement test—was operating at grade level and demonstrated normal social skills.

Fortunately, this family had enough strength to resist my manipulation. I often think of this case and wonder how many of my early prognostications were far off the mark; I suspect a great many. The professional does not have access to all the relevant data. The parent or client knows much more of the really important data to make life decisions, and I have learned, although at times it has been painful to my professional ego, to trust people to make their own decisions. I figure that they know what is best for them.

Humility helps the counselor develop listening skills. Once the counselor recognizes his or her own limitations, he or she can put aside the personal point of view about what the client should do. If we as counselors have a point of view, then listening stops; we listen only for the weakness so as to present our arguments and thus have our point of view prevail. I did not hear Johnny's mother; I thought only that this was a mother who was denying that she had a child with multiple handicaps, and I filtered everything she said through that perception. I did not respond to her concerns or fears or credit her content; instead, we were engaged in an adversarial relationship that did not grow and, more important, did not benefit her child.

Counselor Mistakes

I have made mistakes on many occasions. Usually these errors are not so much failures of commission as failures to capitalize on a very cogent situation and miss the counseling moment. I almost always recover from my insensitivities and gaffes. I bring them up at the next session or, if I am really bothered by them, I call up the client and apologize. These apologies have helped relationships because they convey my humanity and my vulnerability, both of which contribute to client growth (mine too).

The failure to capitalize on situations, however, is a reflection on my lack of skill at the time. I cannot guarantee to clients that I will always be skillful. I can only promise that I will be doing the best I know how to do and will continue to be learning and growing as a professional.

I have observers in the form of practicum students in all my parent groups. After each session, we have a postmortem with an eye to what I might have done differently. I find these sessions helpful, and many times I can recover a mistake, although it is never quite the same as having acted a certain way initially. These are the "should have done's" that I think all professionals carry with them. Early in my career I tape-recorded sessions and listened carefully to the playbacks, which helped me identify areas on which I needed to work. In more than 40 years of doing this, I still find areas on which I need to work. This keeps me going, as I always feel professionally challenged. I guess when I finally do it all right all the time, it will be time for me to retire.

The Unattractive Client

Occasionally I meet a client toward whom it is difficult for me to develop an unconditional positive regard. These clients are like weeds in the garden and bring to mind the Ralph Waldo Emerson quote, "A weed is a plant whose virtues have not yet been discovered." I have to keep searching these "weeds" to find those virtues. I have found that, with care and patience, some of my ugliest weeds have turned into beautiful flowers; some, unfortunately, have remained weeds. If I cannot see them as weeds looking for a place to belong, then I try to see them as a teacher—that usually works. I also try to remember the Dalai Lama's words: "We all seek happiness."

Counseling Caveats

Counseling is often as much a matter of what you don't do as what you actually do. A description of some common pitfalls follows.

Stereotyping

Stereotyping is a seemingly efficient way of putting clients in "little boxes" of characteristics. If we do this long enough, we cease to see who is actually there and respond only to our expectations of them. I strenuously avoid reading any material that purports to describe the characteristics of a cultural or racial minority because it invariably leads to stereotyping. In my experience, no two women, no two African Americans, no two Jews, are exactly alike. This is especially true of parents of children with disabilities. They respond in many different ways to their child's disabilities, and I must put aside my preconceptions when I encounter a new family. For example, some families are cognitively focused and need a great deal of content at the outset in order to feel secure. Thus it is essential to listen carefully to each client right from the beginning in order to be truly culturally sensitive; the client will teach us how to help him or her. We must view each client as a marvelous experiment of one; we are all multicultural.

Transference

Transference is a term borrowed from psychoanalysis and occurs whenever we bring prior experiences into the present; this sets up expectations. Whenever I respond intensely to someone on a first meeting, I stop and consider whether I might be responding from an imprinting in my past. For example, I tend to give 10 extra IQ points to men with mustaches, because my father had a mustache. Such transferences can lead us astray because we cease to see the client as an individual. As I have gotten older, and maybe wiser, I seem to have fewer transferences. My early experiences seem to have less influence on my current perceptions. As we get older, we can free ourselves from our past and reinvent ourselves—this is very encouraging.

Projection

Projection is the attribution of one's own ideas, feelings, values, or attitudes to the client. As with transference, we don't often recognize that we are projecting. It is the ownership problem again. For example, the felt need to refer a client to counseling may reflect my inadequacy, not the client's. Fellow clinicians sometimes ask me, "At what point do you refer a client to counseling?" I respond, "Never. I refer myself." I might tell a client that where we are is currently beyond my scope of practice and I don't wish to continue, but I don't refer the client to counseling. In this situation, many families refer themselves to counseling; others choose not to because it is not in their value system to seek therapy. Referral to counseling reflects *my* values, and not necessarily my client's. For some families, a mental health professional is very threatening, and I need to respect that. Similarly, I'm sometimes asked, "How do you get fathers involved with the nursery?" The answer is, we don't. Some families work quite well without the father's participation, with both parents quite happy in their roles. They may not function as we would or as we would like them to, but they are functioning nonetheless. Projections always lead to a judgmental attitude that severely limits our ability to counsel. We must take families as they are, not try to mold them into what we'd like them to be. Whenever we begin thinking someone *should* do something, we should stop and consider whether we are projecting. We need to abandon our egocentric view of the world and accept people as they are; when we do that, they can grow.

Implicit Expectations

Probably nothing damages relationships more than *implicit expectations*, which are unacknowledged assumptions about the other person's behavior. This problem occurs frequently in parent–professional relationships around the issue of assuming responsibility. Parents often enter into the relationship expecting the therapist to "fix" the child, while the clinician expects a more collaborative relationship where the parent is active in the therapeutic process. If neither party has made its expectations explicit, the relationship will founder on the shoals of failed expectations. Usually in this scenario there is much unexpressed, displaced anger, and there is limited communication between parent and therapist. At the outset, the therapist needs to elicit from clients their expectations and to see if these match the therapist's. The difference may be negotiable and a contract achieved. All my contracts entail some parent involvement. If we cannot agree, I refer families to another facility. Experience has taught me that I cannot be—or, more appropriately, choose not to be—everything to everybody. There are people I choose not to work with because what they seek would violate a professional boundary, and it is best to accept clients whose expectations are within my clinical limitations.

Over-Helping

Over-helping was described earlier as the Annie Sullivan syndrome. If we assume too much responsibility for the clinical outcome, the client can learn helplessness. The more we help people overtly, the less they do, and the fewer opportunities they have to develop their own resources. We give to life what life demands of us. In many instances, adversity is our best teacher because it forces us to develop capacities that might otherwise lie dormant. Clinicians must find the therapeutic equator for helping each family. We must be gentle coaches, helping as covertly as possible and allowing families to take full credit for their successes. Some families will require little assistance; others will require more. As good teachers, we always want to be operating on the periphery of what a family is ready to learn, armed with the assumption and attitude that the family is competent. Our goal is to empower, and we do this best by not over-helping and by being there in a supportive way. Finding the appropriate entry point for each family is what distinguishes the superior clinician from the mediocre one.

Denial Misunderstood

Denial has already been mentioned and will be discussed in the next chapter, but its importance cannot be overemphasized: A misunderstanding of the denial mechanism can seriously compromise the professional–client relationship. When clinicians do not understand the crucial role that denial plays in client welfare, an adversarial relationship often develops. Denial is an emotion-based coping strategy derived from fear. To the insensitive clinician, it may seem that the client or the family is not following through on good recommendations, which may generate anger on the part of the clinician. An admonitory lecture usually follows, which in turn leads to passive-aggressive behavior on the client's part. The clinician needs to look deeper into the client's behavior and see the anxiety that is motivating it. People cannot be pushed out of denial; they give it up when they feel able to cope in a more proactive way. Empowerment leads to the abatement of denial, and that's where the clinician's therapeutic focus needs to be.

Cheerleading

As helping professionals, we want to take away pain. Unfortunately, most of the disorders we deal with create irreversible pain that cannot be eradicated; to try to do so invalidates the client's experience. We are telling clients that they have no right to their feelings, and even though we might temporarily make them feel better, the pain of loss will return—and then they will feel guilty. It is best to sit and listen compassionately with clients in pain, thereby acknowledging and validating their experience. People have their own marvelous capacity to make themselves feel better.

The following anonymously written piece, I think, says it all about counseling:

> When I ask you to listen to me and you start giving advice you have not done what I asked.
>
> When I ask you to listen to me and you begin to tell me why I shouldn't feel that way you are trampling on my feelings.
>
> When I ask you to listen to me and you feel you have to do something to solve my problem, you have failed me, strange as that may seem.
>
> Listen! All I asked was that you listen, not talk or do—just hear me.
>
> Advice is cheap: 10 cents will get you both Dear Abby and Billy Graham in the same newspaper.
>
> And I can do for myself; I'm not helpless. Maybe discouraged and faltering, but not helpless.
>
> When you do something for me that I can and need to do for myself, you contribute to my fear and weakness.
>
> But, when you accept as a simple fact that I do feel what I feel, no matter how irrational, then I can quit trying to convince you and can get about the business of understanding what's behind this irrational feeling. And when that's clear, the answers are obvious and I don't need advice. Irrational feelings make sense when we understand what's behind them. Perhaps that's why prayer works, sometimes, for some people because God is mute, and He doesn't give advice or try to fix things. "They" just listen and let you work it out for yourself.
>
> So, please listen and just hear me. And, if you want to talk, wait a minute for your turn, and I'll listen to you.

THE GROUP PROCESS

At the outset of this chapter, I would like to share my very strong bias in favor of group counseling. I feel that group sessions are an efficacious means of counseling; in fact, I seldom do formal individual counseling. Within an individual session, I have to be very wise and very alert; there is no help. Within the group setting, many resources are available and, although I act as leader, I do not have to be so all-encompassing; invariably when I am at a loss, someone in the group rescues me. I think that within a group there is marvelous health, strength, and a collective wisdom that supersedes the wisdom of any one member. The task of the leader is to unleash that wisdom.

My group work has been mainly with parents of children with hearing impairment. I have, however, had some experience with parents of children with other handicaps, groups of hard-of-hearing adults, multiple sclerosis spouse groups, smoking cessation groups for the American Cancer Society, student clinician groups, and groups of practicing speech–language pathologists and audiologists.

Groups in Speech–Language Pathology and Audiology

It is difficult to determine from reading the literature on communication disorders just how extensively groups are used. I suspect they are used much more frequently than the literature would indicate. There appear to be two types of groups: communication therapy groups and counseling groups. The therapy group composed of individuals with speech–language disorders is used fairly frequently and has a long history. This type of group is convened to work on a specific speech or language problem. Over 50 years ago, Backus and Beasley (1951) found that results from group therapy with children with speech disorders were superior to results from individual therapy. Albertini, Smith, and Metz (1983) found that deaf adolescents did as well working on their speech within a group as did a control group that had individual therapy. In the years between these two reports, many others were published that supported the notion of group therapy if for no other reason than better use of therapist time. I suspect that many therapy groups are started and maintained in the hope of reducing a therapist's waiting list.

My concern here is the counseling group (not to imply that counseling is not part of a therapy group), which may or may not be composed of individuals who have speech–language disorders. This group has an implicit mandate to deal with feelings. (In practice, I suspect, many counseling groups stay with content because of the therapists' insecurity.) The groups are convened and conceived as places where individuals can talk about the feelings generated by having speech–language disabilities or having relatives who have speech–language disabilities. Counseling has been used in a variety of group contexts, such as with parents of children with speech defects (E. Webster, 1968, 1977), parents of deaf children (Dee, 1981), spouses of aphasic patients (Bardach, 1969; Emerson, 1980), stroke patients (Singler, 1982), deaf adults (Schein, 1982), and stutterers (Ginsberg & Wexler, 1999). Apparently these groups are used quite frequently with varying degrees of success, depending on how well the group can overcome the communication problem.

Counseling groups are also used extensively outside of the field of communication disorders. Seligman (1982) reported on group counseling for special populations, including cancer patients, people with physical disabilities, elderly individuals, drug abusers, prison populations, people with mental retardation, people with visual impairments, and alcoholics. Groups have also been used extensively with people who have chronic illness (Cole, O'Conner, & Bennett, 1979; Davies, Priddy, & Tinkleberg, 1986; Hinkle, 1991; McKelvey & Borgersen, 1990). Nuland (1994), for example, underscored the healing properties of groups for the families of people with Alzheimer's disease:

> In the case of Alzheimer's disease, it is rarely the patient who recognizes the need for company in the journey through travail. But there is probably no disability of our time in which the presence of support groups can help so decisively to ensure the emotional survival of the closest witness to the disintegration. . . . There is strength in numbers, even when the numbers are only one or two understanding people who can soften the anguish by the simple act of listening. (p. 106)

Probably the most extensive use of group techniques has been in the field of psychotherapy. The definitive text in group psychotherapy to date was written by Yalom (1975), who identified 11 interdependent curative factors in group therapy. I think that eight of these factors (listed below) have wide applicability in counseling groups within the communication disorders field. (I think the three other curative factors that Yalom lists—the development of socialization techniques, imitative behavior, and the corrective recapitulation of the primary family group—either are contained within previous factors or are more appropriate for psychotherapeutic groups.)

Curative Factors in Groups

Instillation of Hope

I personally have an almost mystical belief in the power of the group for healing and growth. By seeing how others have improved, the clients can feel hope for themselves. There is always someone in a group who has overcome adversity, which lifts the spirits of the others. In fact, faith and hope may be the only curative factors one needs, as evidenced by the efficacy of faith healers and placebo therapy. The faith of the therapist in the group process is also transmitted to the clients.

Universality

The group helps individuals recognize that they are not alone in their feelings and perceptions. The parents of a child with a disability often feel that they are crazy or sick for feeling a particular way (which usually involves wishing the child were dead), and when they find out that other parents have felt the same way, they feel relief: They are not alone, and they are not crazy. Universality—a feeling that you can get only within a group format—is very much a factor in dealing with the existential issue of loneliness.

Imparting of Information

Information is provided not only by the leader, although many groups are structured so that the leader provides most of the content, but also by the other members of the group. I am always astonished at how much clients already know. Sometimes some of the least articulate members in the group come up with marvelous, unique solutions. I am also struck by how rarely advice is directly beneficial to a group member, although it is frequently offered within the group. Advice, I think, is the indirect conveyance of a mutual interest and caring, and as such serves a vital function in the group. Of much more lasting value, however, is the knowledge gained from the sharing of experiences. All groups should and almost always do leave the participants more informed than when the group started.

Altruism

By imparting information, group participants get a chance to help one another. People with disabilities rarely have the chance to help anyone, which diminishes their self-esteem. The group situation enables them to receive help without a concomitant loss of self-esteem because the help is reciprocal.

Within the group, members offer support, reassurance, and insights to one another. I have found, for example, that parents of children with disabilities listen much more attentively to another parent than they do to me. Another parent has a credibility that I can never duplicate. A frequent result of a successful counseling group is the desire—and the translation of that desire into action—to help similarly disabled populations. This is a healthy result that has the potential to move the participants away from an almost morbid self-absorption and allow them to grow.

Interpersonal Learning

Human survival depends on the ability to live in groups. Yet I find that many people with whom I come in contact (parents of children with disabilities, student clinicians, speech–language pathologists, audiologists) have poor interpersonal skills, in part, I think, because of poor early learning in their family of origin. They have difficulty communicating with others, being trusting and honest with others, and learning to love more fully. None of this is pathological in the sense that these people are nonfunctional; however, better developed interpersonal skills would enable them to get more joy and satisfaction out of all of their interpersonal interactions. The group can be a very safe vehicle for the participants to enhance their interpersonal learning. They can learn (or, more appropriately, *relearn*) how to be more open and accepting of others, and can then take this knowledge from the group context into their other relationships.

Group Cohesiveness

Cohesiveness, a basic property of groups, is very difficult to define and grasp, yet I think it is an integral factor in successful counseling. Analogous to the relationship in individual therapy, cohesiveness is not a curative factor per se, but rather a precondition. Cohesiveness is related to the attractiveness of the group to its members. I know a group will be successful when I can hardly wait for the sessions to start and I look forward to seeing the other members of the group. Cohesiveness is intricately tied to trust: Where trust develops, much as in individual therapy, groups come together and growth can occur. Whenever someone in a group reveals a deep secret that is accepted and amplified by other members of the group, there is a quantum leap in group cohesiveness.

Another intangible factor, an interpersonal attraction that may or may not occur, also determines cohesiveness. Some groups seem to come together very easily, and I do not have to work for cohesiveness. The members of these groups are attracted to one another because of similar values and, I suspect, some transferences that they bring to the experience. The chemistry in these groups seems right; there is a good mix of talkers and listeners, and individuals like each other. In other groups, cohesiveness is hard to come by—members do not especially like each other or share much with each other. I tend to want to blame the lack of cohesiveness on bad group chemistry and not on my lack of skill. When pressed to the wall, however, I admit a skill issue: I need to pay more careful attention to building trust and cohesiveness in the early stages with groups and to quickly identify when a group is not developing them.

Although I think individuals can and do learn even when a group is not cohesive, I think that the learning is greater and much deeper in a cohesive group. Many of my lifelong and close friendships have developed from being in groups with high degrees of cohesiveness.

Catharsis

Catharsis, which is closely related to universality, is the expression of the considerable affect that surrounds communication disorders. Almost all participants bring to the group pent-up emotions that they have had no safe place to express. The group can provide the vehicle for the release and sharing of these feelings. Families of stroke victims, for example, invariably come to feel that they can talk in the group because they can be understood. Professional groups tend to bring individuals' feelings of inadequacy to the fore, and there is a great deal of relief in being able to express them and to be heard and understood by the other group members.

Catharsis per se is not a curative factor; simply expressing a feeling is not sufficient to promote growth. It is, however, a preliminary to being able to un-hook the feelings from the unhealthy behavior.

Existential Issues

Existential issues are described in detail in Chapter 2. Groups give individuals a chance to work through their questions regarding the issues of death/ life en-hancement, responsibility assumption/dependency, loneliness/love, and mean-inglessness/commitment. Almost all of the personal growth that emerges in the groups I lead can be classified under these existential issues. They are a powerful way of looking at individuals and judging personal growth. When groups, and the individuals within groups, are willing to face the existential issues, then growth and change begin.

Group Goals in Communication Disorders

Yalom's (1975) 11 curative factors can all be subsumed under three broad cat-egories that relate to the goals of groups within the field of communication dis-orders: conveying content, sharing of affect, and personal growth. The goals are contained within the curative factors and need only be discussed briefly here as they relate to communication disorders.

Content

All groups to a certain extent have a content mandate; that is, the convening of the group makes possible the sharing of information and experiences of the members. Learning is unavoidable within a group context, although sometimes what is learned is what the leader neither expected nor intended. Groups, I think, proceed best when the leader is not perceived as the sole source of content. This may violate expectations of the group members, but in the long run, I think that more is learned from the group experience when there is a collective responsibility to teach one another. Unfortunately, many groups within the field of communication disorders seem to have content dissemination as their sole purpose, and usually this content is supplied by the professional. These groups are missing much.

Affect Release

Being the parent of a child with a disability, having an important family member undergo a catastrophic illness, or having a communication disorder will engender a great many feelings that usually have no healthy way of being expressed. Frequently the feelings—especially anger—are repressed, which results in depression, or are displaced to others, which impairs interpersonal relationships. The group can become the means for releasing the affect in a safe environment among people who understand those feelings. The group, more than any other vehicle I know, can give sanction and permission to its members to experience their feelings.

Personal Growth

Personal growth is not ordinarily thought of as a responsibility within the discipline of communication disorders, yet I feel that we must address this issue in order to be more effective as professionals. For example, we need to help parents of children with disabilities become more assertive and less compliant when participating with professionals in making educational plans for their child. For this to happen, the parents (as well as all people with communication disorders) need to have high self-esteem and a more internal locus of control. People with communication disorders have to learn to take responsibility for their disabilities in order to minimize the negative effects on their personal lives. They may learn ways of utilizing their disorders to help others, such as when they form self-help groups and political action groups to further benefit persons with disabilities in our society.

A group can serve as a powerful personal growth vehicle by allowing individuals to help others, and if the leader is willing to "sit on his or her wisdom," the group members can take control and, therefore, learn responsibility assumption. This cannot help but carry over into their everyday lives.

Leadership

The leadership of the group is a vital factor in determining the group's success. Groups are entities unto themselves; that is, each group has a unique personality, and no two groups are ever the same. The principles underlying successful individual counseling are equally applicable to counseling within a group setting. The counselor must treat the group from a humanistic point of view, with acceptance, genuineness, empathy, and concern. The leader must be seen as a caring person.

Yalom (1975), in his exhaustive study of encounter groups, found four leadership functions that were directly related to outcomes:

1. *Emotional stimulation*—accomplished by confronting, modeling, risk-taking, and disclosing self.

2. *Caring*—accomplished by offering support, affection, warmth, concern, and genuineness.

3. *Meaning attribution*—accomplished by exploring, clarifying, interpreting, and providing a cognitive framework for change.

4. *Executive function*—accomplished by setting limits and rules, managing time, and suggesting procedures. (p. 477)

Lieberman, Yalom, and Miles (1973) found that those leaders who were very high in caring and meaning attribution and who were moderate in emotional stimulation and executive function were the most successful leaders and that their successes were independent of their theoretical orientations. Groups grew with leaders who cared about them and who could provide members with a cognitive framework for understanding their behavior. Groups were limited in their growth by leaders who were too high or too low in provoking feelings and in executive function. Too little executive function tended to create confused groups, whereas too much tended to create passive groups. Too little emotional stimulation led to devitalized groups, whereas emotionally overcharged groups were chaotic.

In my experience with parent groups in particular, I have found that it is seldom necessary to provide emotional stimulation. The affect is so high to begin with that, when the group provides a safe, caring atmosphere, the feelings emerge without any need to provoke the affect.

The most important function of the leader is to set norms for the group. These are the implicit and sometimes very explicit rules by which the group is to function. A group's norms are established very early and are very hard to change once established. The leader establishes the norms by modeling and, especially with procedural norms, by stating them explicitly. The most frequently used mechanism for establishing norms in the group is the reinforcement paradigm. The leader, by virtue of the power accorded by the members of the group, uses social approval as a powerful reinforcement agent to ensure group norms. Thus, those behaviors or remarks chosen to be acknowledged tend to become valued by the group, and those behaviors that are not acknowledged tend to be devalued. Most leaders reinforce norms unwittingly, based on some deep-seated and unconscious prejudices that they have.

I think my greatest source of failure with groups has been in allowing unhealthy group norms to develop and in not acting soon enough to prevent a poor norm from taking hold. In one group that I was leading, I was called away to answer the phone (something I no longer allow to happen), and when I returned the parents were having a passionate discussion on which was the best diaper to use on their children. I listened for a while and then very stupidly confronted the group as to why they were wasting their group time discussing such a trivial topic when they could do that elsewhere. The group thereafter became a very low-risk, low-contributing group, one of the dullest groups I ever worked with. When I was finally able to see what was happening (2 months later—I am a bit slow), I realized that I had established a norm of leader-generated topics. Apparently, as far as the group was concerned, only certain topics were appropriate to discuss within the meeting, and they had to guess what was acceptable because if they did not, they would incur my wrath. The best strategy for them to adopt was to play safe and not risk a new topic. The topics groups select to discuss are never irrelevant; however, leaders sometimes are.

This group never recovered. If I had it to do over again (a lament most professionals share), I would say, "It must be so hard for you when you have so many choices." This remark might have moved the group to look at all the choices they had to make regarding their children. At the very least, I would have done better to have kept quiet and allowed some other members to point out how they were wasting time. In either case, I do not think that I would have had a dull group.

Interaction Norm

If group members are to relate and learn from one another, then they have to interact among themselves. Most groups begin with a question directed toward the leader. If the question is answered, another question-and-answer exchange is usually encouraged. This means that the leader can get trapped into providing content via answering the questions and speaking about 50% of the time.

If the group is to function as a group, the leader has to quickly get away from answering questions and encourage interactions among all the group members. I feel that if I take up no more than 10% of the group's time by talking, it is usually a successful group. The interaction norm allows for the sharing of information and for the helping that can occur among members.

Initiative Norm

I think the initiative norm is vital for growth: The group members must learn that if they want something to happen, they must make it happen. I come into the group with no agenda and no topic. The topics will be determined by the group, and if the members wish to sit and be passive, nothing happens. Early in the history of a group, a silence descends while the group waits to be told what to do and how to proceed. If the leader takes control at this juncture, a norm of a leader-controlled group is established. Once this happens, the members become spectators; the leader can become very resentful about doing all the work. It is very hard for a professional not to take initiative, however, because it conforms to the implicit expectations of both the professional and the client. I almost never use structured experiences early in the life of a group because it establishes a leader-initiated group.

Self-Disclosure

Self-disclosure is a necessary component of growth. It is hard for me to see how group participants can learn if they are unwilling to share themselves. I must establish a group norm whereby individuals, when they do reveal, are never penalized and are always supported. Self-disclosure must always be safe, especially when a participant finally reveals his or her guilty secret. A parent group will become very cohesive when another parent can say, "I always felt that way," or when other members will accept the secret without saying or implying that the group member should not feel that way. When there are many "shoulds" floating around, groups become very inhibited and little self-disclosure occurs.

In one group I facilitated, a laryngectomized man revealed for the first time that he never used his artificial larynx when he went outside because it embarrassed him. None of the other group members told him that he "should" use his larynx. Instead they listened and expressed to him their understanding of how hard it was to appear so deviant. After a while he began crying and received a great deal of emotional support from the group. Several sessions later he announced that he had begun using the larynx in public.

Self-disclosure is never forced. Participants need to feel free not to reveal themselves if they so desire (which is actually another norm in itself).

One way that the leader can encourage self-disclosure is by revealing him- or herself, which can be tricky because the timing must be rather precise. Early in the group's life, an important issue is the leader's credibility. If the leader's guilty secrets are revealed too soon, that credibility might be sacrificed. Self-disclosure by the leader can be very helpful for the group because it helps dispel the authority issue. Clients can see that professionals are human and sometimes need the help that the group can provide. I am, however, very reluctant to self-disclose too early in the life of the group, and expect that the self-disclosure norm will develop spontaneously from the emotional need for validation and from the trust and acceptance norms that begin to develop.

Confrontation

It is vital that group members learn to "check out" with one another when they are concerned about something. Many problems in interpersonal relationships occur from making assumptions without any checks on reality. For example, a student who assumed I was angry with her because I did not smile when we met could operate on that assumption to the detriment of our relationship. If, however, we had established a confrontation norm, the student would feel free to question me on how I felt about her, and might find that I had been preoccupied with some personal problems and that my not smiling was not a reflection on how I felt about her. If in fact I was angry with her, then we would have had an opportunity to discuss what was interfering in our relationship. In either event, we would both win from the confrontation.

I can relax in a group once a confrontation norm has been established because it means that my behavior and statements will not be misunderstood or go unquestioned: The participants will test reality with me and with each other if need be.

The confrontation norm is best established by role modeling. The leader must select an appropriate time to demonstrate this behavior. Confrontation requires a great deal of group trust and is frightening to members.

Unfortunately, this norm is not common in many interpersonal relationships, and participants are usually fearful when confrontations occur. Confrontation is closely related to self-disclosure because all confrontation involves a disclosure of self in regard to another person. Self-disclosure generally emerges first because it is safer to talk only about oneself than it is to talk about oneself in relation to someone else who is present. The same conditions that lead a group to self-disclosure also lead to developing a confrontation norm.

Confrontation is not necessarily about negative feelings; one can also confront others with feelings of warmth and liking. I find, however, that the first confrontation feelings to emerge are very often anger and resentment. Unfortunately, most people are less threatened by expressing angry feelings than they are by expressing loving feelings.

Here-and-Now Norm

Probably nothing is deadlier in a group than having members tell long anecdotes to which nobody else has access; interest in the group diminishes rapidly. The facilitator has to find immediacy in the material and bring it to the present. Thus, to a participant relating a story in which he had a dispute with the hearing-aid dealer, for example, I might respond, "What did you do with your anger?" (inviting self-disclosure) and then, "Have you been angry with me?" (inviting confrontation). The more immediate the experience is, the more exciting it is, and the greater the potential for its being a learning experience for everyone. When it is material to which everyone has access, as in recalling an event that happened in one of the group meetings, all the members of the group can contribute and receive and give feedback.

A here-and-now norm is established by timely interventions on the facilitator's part that force the group member into the present. Groups will not start out with a here-and-now orientation as they have no group history from which to work. Participants have to reveal themselves and establish their credibility. There also needs to be some elapsed time for interactions among members to be processed. Here-and-now is a powerful norm directed toward achieving the goals of personal growth because it encourages interpersonal interaction within the group.

Respecting Individual Needs

Group norms, if not watched, can become very restrictive, especially when they promote a high degree of conformity It is not healthy for everyone to adhere rigidly to a particular established norm. Individuals need to feel that they have control over their own behaviors and that learning will proceed when they are ready. One of the few explicit norms I establish in every group I lead is that the participants do not have to talk if they do not wish to, and that no question must be answered. When a group decision is required, it is necessary to arrive at a compromise or willingness for the dissenters to agree to conform to the norm. For example, I cannot tolerate being in rooms with a lot of cigarette smoke, and I prefer that there be no smoking in the group. I tell this to the group at our first session and then talk to the smokers (nowadays it is hard to find any smokers). I try to respect their felt need to smoke and ask if they are willing to go the length of the session without smoking. If not, I offer a smoking break to the group in which we all stop for several minutes.

My willingness to negotiate and to discuss the issue with the smokers sends the important message to the group that I try to respect each individual's needs. If I entered a group with the statement that smoking is not permitted, I would be establishing a leader-dominated group in which my needs superseded other members' needs. The time taken to negotiate the smoking issue is well spent; it establishes a powerful group norm. Such seemingly little things can determine the success of the group.

Procedural Norms

Procedural norms determine how the group will function. There are usually a number of givens over which the group has no control, such as number of sessions and length of time of each session. I am always very clear at the outset about how much time is available. If time is a negotiable issue with the group, I enter into negotiation during the first session so that everyone knows the length of their time commitment and agrees to it. I also am sure to be at the group meetings on time and end all meetings at the agreed-upon hour.

I try to establish a norm of confidentiality in almost all counseling groups that I lead. I know I cannot impose confidentiality as I have no way of enforcing it. I tell the group that I will not talk about the group with any outsiders and that I hope they will do the same. I do not allow casual visitors to the group. In my academic classes, I do not talk about confidentiality in initial sessions because confidentiality implies (or almost imposes) a self-disclosure norm on a group. If a group of students begins to self-disclose, I then talk to them about confidentiality and see if we can come to some consensus.

Stages of Group Development

Although each group is unique, all groups seem to develop along similar lines. A group facilitator needs to have a sense of the developmental sequence of groups to be able to diagnose quickly when a group is functioning deviantly and to perhaps provide some corrective measures. Almost invariably the difficulty is caused by an unhealthy group norm that is limiting group growth. Virtually no controlled research studies on group development have been published; what do exist are mainly nonsystematic clinical observations (Yalom, 1975).

The Group at Inception

I usually start groups by introducing myself, explaining how I came to be there, and telling what expectations I have for myself in the group. I then invite the members to introduce themselves and describe why they are there. After everyone has finished, I mention any procedural norms (time of sessions, smoking, the right to not answer questions, etc.). These are kept to a minimum, as most norms are developed as a function of how I behave and which group behaviors I will reinforce. Next, I might remark that I hope that everyone will come to value the experience. At this point usually a loud silence ensues, which seems to be eternal but is probably no more than 30 seconds in duration. Almost invariably the silence is broken by a question directed at me, which is usually a procedural-type question as the members begin to look to the leader to provide them with structure. For example, a participant might ask, "What are we supposed to do here?" to which I usually respond, "What would you like to do here?"

At inception, the group is primarily engaged in developing structure and establishing credibility. When the members begin to learn that I will not structure the session, they start to act and, in acting, reveal themselves. Everybody is still on their best "cocktail party" behavior; a parent group might begin with one parent telling the story about discovering her child's disability, which establishes her credentials to be in the group, and invariably provokes other members to start telling their stories. When they find nods of acceptance and a matching of experiences, cohesiveness starts to build. Usually a lot of affect is expressed. The beginning stages of a parent group are usually very cathartic as the parents reveal the pent-up feelings that have not previously been expressed.

A student group or a working professional group usually starts out very hesitantly with long, embarrassed silences. The members are not sure how to proceed and are uncertain how much of themselves they are willing to reveal. Usually there is someone in the group who is desperate enough to risk some self-disclosure. If that is accepted, an intimacy spiral begins to develop, and more and more self-disclosures occur. Professional groups have generally been the most emotionally muted groups I have worked with. Often this happens when there is a hierarchical structure to the group, such as students and supervisors, or employees and employers; mobilizing these groups requires enormous amounts of patience. These groups may also have a hidden agenda; there is a history of relationships about which the leader has no knowledge, and there are potential traps. Leaders very often are scapegoated by these groups for bringing into the open very painful topics that the group has preferred to ignore.

For example, I once worked with the staff of a school for the deaf. After two very dull sessions punctuated with long silences, the group members began to open up. It soon developed that a great deal of hostility was directed toward one teacher who was chronically late to class and was not, as viewed by the other teachers, very competent. I was able to get them to specify this teacher by not accepting generalizations such as, "Some teachers are always late." I asked them who they had in mind and when they finally specified one teacher, everyone jumped on the bandwagon and the accused teacher left in a gush of tears. The group then turned on me and accused me of causing all this. The group never became a comfortable place for the members to reveal more about themselves, and it certainly was not a comfortable place for me. I think the group and I learned much from that encounter, and I think the school ultimately benefited by that teacher's resignation. It is much easier to work with a group of strangers who have no history together, because then the leader is always privy to the developing history of the group.

Almost no confrontation occurs in beginning stages of group development because there is insufficient trust. Invariably, confrontation stems from the leader's role-modeling this behavior, which needs to occur at a somewhat later point in group development. A classic dilemma for the group leader occurs when a member of a beginning group is starting to establish destructive norms for the group and nobody is willing to confront the person. For example, in a recent student group, one participant kept monopolizing the group with long, boring anecdotes that bore no relationship to what anyone else had been saying. She filled every silence, and commandeered the gaps between silences. Nobody in the group seemed confident enough to challenge her. I took responsibility for pointing out her behavior and solicited feedback from other members as to how they were feeling about her. My intervention came too soon in the group's development, because the "monopolizer" stopped attending regularly, and when she did attend, she seldom spoke. She denied being fearful of speaking but seemed to lose all interest in the group. The rest of the group, however, became even more fearful, afraid that I might put them on the "hot seat." The group became a very low-risk, low-participation group characterized by long uncomfortable silences and very little self-disclosure. Group members no longer saw me as a support. Even though I solicited feedback about how they felt about the incident and about me, the group never became cohesive.

In retrospect, I realize that I needed to wait longer before confronting the monopolizer in this group; I did not allow the group time to learn to act cohesively. Groups need time to develop sufficient trust: Familiarity breeds liking when we can get below the surface behavior. I have found it a mistake to try to push groups in the early stages of development; they operate in an unfolding process. The timing of a confrontation presents a dilemma for the group facilitator, because waiting too long is equally destructive to the group process. In one parent group I was working with, a deaf mother of a deaf child would not let the other mothers grieve about their children's deafness. Every time they tried to say something negative about deafness, the deaf mother would say, "But look at me," meaning that she was functioning as a wife and mother and had made a good adjustment to her deafness. Meanwhile, the other parents were only seeing that her speech was virtually unintelligible and she needed an interpreter to function in the group; they were still very much in the denial/resistance stages of coping. It was a problem that I never really solved. The group was very restricted and needed to be confronted by the group leader, but I never found what seemed to me a satisfactory time to confront the group. I think I lacked the professional courage at that time to challenge the group to open up to what was happening. This was one of my less successful groups, and I think I learned much from it. Unfortunately, our clients often suffer from our learning.

Resistance to the group process also begins to develop early. The resistance usually manifests itself in the group members' focusing on differences among them. The parent groups that I lead at Emerson College are composed of parents of young deaf children, parents of children with normal hearing, student clinicians, and sometimes a practicing clinician who wants to learn more about groups. The professionals and I meet after the group session to process the experience. Almost invariably, the professionals and students have a low level of participation in the group. They feel that it is a parent group and they have little to contribute. As they become more comfortable, however, they begin to see the commonalities between themselves and the parents, and frequently use the group as a valuable personal growth vehicle.

The Working Group

The developmental stages of a group are rarely well demarcated. There is no single point at which a group announces that it is ready to move from the inception stage to the working stage. This stage is characterized by cohesiveness, by conflict, and by redefining the leader.

It might seem contradictory to say that the group is both cohesive and in conflict, but these attributes are not incompatible. Only when one feels safe within a relationship can one afford to be confrontational. Conflict, when it emerges within the group, is usually a marker of the level of cohesiveness within the group. In initial stages, everyone is on his or her best behavior, uncertain as to the safety of the situation. When the members feel secure, they confront. Usually the confrontation is with an outsider, as when parents accuse the student clinicians of not having a child and therefore not being able to understand them. If no obvious outsider exists, then the behavior is directed toward the leader for somehow failing them. (The leader in one sense is always an outsider, and very often being group facilitator means that the leader has to continually confront existential aloneness.)

When the group moves into its working stage, it is ready to redefine the leader and settle into its working structure. Anger is directed toward me because I will not tell the group what to do, and parents wonder if I could possibly understand them, as I do not have a child with a disability. Conflict cannot be eliminated from, human interaction; we grow from conflict. It is the resolution of the conflict that determines the group structure. We negotiate among ourselves, we compromise, and we develop the mechanisms that enable us to attend to tasks.

Content also becomes very valuable and is readily transferred among the members. A good working group is characterized by a joint knowledge of the strengths and weaknesses of each member and an ability to utilize the talent that is in the group. The topics that appeared in the initial stages of the group now reappear and are discussed in more detail and from a different perspective. Thus, some participants who said little the first time around may become very vocal (the previous discussion may have set them to thinking about the issue when they were not ready to share). Other members may have rethought their positions. I find with parent groups in particular that all the cogent issues emerge in the first few sessions and no new topics occur thereafter. It is a recycling process. A richness and complexity are generated by the interactions of the group members, and groups never run out of things to say.

In a well-functioning group, the trust level is high, and when conflict does emerge, it is dealt with openly. Positive feelings among the members emerge, and some are even directed toward the leader, who is now accepted as a working member of the group. I realize I am portraying an idealized vision of the working group. Not all of the groups I have dealt with achieve this level of functioning—many get close, but unfortunately some groups never do. Nevertheless, I have never failed to learn from a group.

The Terminating Group

Termination is an integral part of the group process and is not to be trivialized or minimized. The process of termination itself becomes an impetus to further growth. My own death-avoidance issues have very often interfered with providing a group a satisfactory termination ritual. Groups need time and space to tie up loose ends (there are always loose ends) and to mourn their demise. Often the group avoids the task of termination because it is very painful. The leader can use that termination awareness as a spur to complete work. I try to keep groups working until the last possible moment. Often groups will start the termination process too soon; if I allow this to happen, some good work can be lost. The leader must exercise a timing judgment.

I have terminated groups by suggesting that each member take a moment to reflect on the group experience and to imagine going home. I ask, "What messages do you wish you had delivered? What 'I should have saids' do you think you might have?" I then suggest that we spend the rest of the session delivering the messages. Yalom (1975) said the following about the termination process:

> Throughout, the therapist facilitates the group work by disclosing his own feelings about separation. The therapist, no less than the patients, will miss the group. For him, too, it has been a place of anguish, conflict, fear, and also of great beauty; some of life's truest and most poignant moments occur in the small and yet limitless microcosm of the therapy group. (p. 374)

Other Considerations

Use of Structured Experiences

Structured experiences are generally any activities, usually leader generated, that are designed to accelerate the group process. They are techniques that encourage self-disclosure or bypass the conventional social restrictions. For example, a new group may be divided into dyads in which each member of the dyad interviews the other. When the group reconvenes, each member of the dyad introduces the other to the group. There are many such devices to help the group through the initial introductory stage.

The problem with leader-directed exercises is that they do not encourage initiative by group members. They tend to create a passive group that sits back and waits for the leader to give the next exercise. The exercises can become an excuse for an individual's behavior and can limit responsibility assumption. Exercises frequently are used to rescue a group (actually, the leader) and in the long term are seldom helpful. Lieberman et al. (1973) found that the group leaders who used exercises most frequently were regarded by the members of their groups as more competent, more effective, and more perceptive than leaders who used structured experiences sparingly. Yet, and very much to the point, the members of the groups that had the most highly structured experiences had the poorest outcomes (i.e., fewer positive changes and less ability to maintain positive change over time) than the less structured groups.

I have used and still occasionally use structured experiences in my workshops. I use them sparingly, and they need to fit organically within the flow of the group process. When effective, they occur or seem to occur spontaneously. In a previous book (Luterman, 1979), I devoted an entire chapter to structured experience. These activities include role playing, hypothetical families, and guided fantasies. Although I have had positive feedback from readers who have used them to advantage, I am always a bit uncomfortable with their use. I feel that they can get a group and group leader into trouble that they may not yet be prepared to handle. Although structured experiences can be valuable if used judiciously, they also can open members of a group before the group is ready, and they seem to encourage a technique orientation for the group leader that I do not like

Homogeneity of Grouping

The general tendency to keep groups homogeneous is usually reflected in the diagnostic label. Thus, there are groups of laryngectomized persons, stutterers, families of stroke victims, and so on. When I began working with groups, I restricted the groups to parents of young deaf children who had no other disabilities. I was trying for a very homogeneous group, as I did not feel secure enough at that time to handle any additional problems presented by outlier parents. I soon learned that homogeneity is a myth. Even though the group shared the same diagnostic label, there were enormous differences between and among the members. There were differences in education, values, and child-rearing practices. In fact, an early manifestation of resistance to the group process was the pointing out of the many differences that existed among the members (e.g., "They can't possibly understand me because my child is hard of hearing and their children are deaf"). One primary task of the facilitator is to focus the group members on their similarities (e.g., by asking, "Can you tell me some ways in which you are like these other people?").

As I have become more secure in my abilities, I have allowed more obviously heterogeneous groupings to occur. I began letting into the group parents of children with multiple disabilities and hearing impairment, parents of older deaf children, and parents of normally hearing children. Recently, I have worked with groups of parents of children of mixed disabilities. Each time I have increased the apparent heterogeneity of the group, the group has become the richer for it. Parents of hearing children have added a commonality to the child-rearing problems, parents of older deaf children have added their experience, and parents of children with other disabilities have led to the appreciation of the universality of the experience of parenting a child with a disability. These different parents have stretched me professionally, and I now welcome and encourage diversity in my groups.

Group Size and Setting

Generally the groups I work with have between 8 and 15 members. I find that this is a good working group size because there are enough members for sufficient interactions among the participants, and not so many members as to require inordinate amounts of time for members to establish their credibility. Larger groups take much longer to establish trust. I also do not allow new people to join the group except at clear demarcation points, such as semester breaks. New members tend to hold back the group development, as the group requires time to absorb the newcomer and to reestablish cohesiveness. It also takes time for the new member to figure out the group norms.

I always try to hold meetings in a comfortable room and to have the participants sit in a circle. Thus, members and the leader can establish eye contact with each other and can read one another's body language. Chairs also need to be comfortable, as the duration of most groups is 1 to 2 hours. A professor of mine once said that the mind can absorb only as much as the seat can endure.

Filling the Available Time

The duration of a group is usually arbitrarily determined. The exigencies of calendar, finances, and participant availability seem to have more bearing on group length than does the amount of therapeutic progress. In one sense, groups are never finished; they are always in the process of becoming, and new material is always emerging. In this way, they are not unlike human beings. For me, the group meeting is a magical moment to be enjoyed and savored for that time and never to be replicated.

Groups have a marvelous way of filling the available time. There is a subconscious and, I think, collective knowledge as to how far a group can go together on a journey. Carl Rogers was once asked, "How far can you get with nondirective therapy when you have only 20 minutes time?" His reputed response was, "Twenty minutes worth." I have had some wonderfully intense group experiences that lasted a total of 2 hours. These groups are almost like a speeded-up motion picture. We all knew that we had only 2 hours to work, so all the trivialities were eliminated, cohesiveness developed very quickly, and self-disclosure was high. Several of my most satisfying professional experiences have occurred in groups with a very short life span.

The counseling group can have a tremendous value in the therapeutic process. It can be used for the families of individuals with communicative disorders as a supplement to individual therapy, or it can be combined with therapy sessions. Groups can be used very flexibly. Developing skills in facilitating groups should be part of a speech–language therapist's or audiologist's training. I think there is no greater gift that we can give to our clients than a well-facilitated support group.

WORKING WITH FAMILIES

Family has always been very important to me. I am part of a second-generation immigrant family; none of my grandparents could speak English very well. Since we were aliens in an alien land, we were forced to rely on each other because as individuals we were not yet comfortable with the dominant culture. My father would tell us children frequently, "Blood is thicker than water," meaning that we could rely on family more then we could on nonfamily. When one of us moved, we all moved. I grew up with an extended family of grandparents, aunts, uncles, and cousins all living within a mile of each other. From the perspective of 70-odd years, I now see that we were an enmeshed family.

That family injunction of "Blood is thicker than water," which is buried deep within my psyche, has carried over to my professional life. After working for several years as a clinical audiologist, I began to feel increasingly uncomfortable with the restricted and limited involvement I had with clients and their families. I remember vividly a clinical experience in which I knew I was "short." (This is another "nugget of gold" situation based on "sins" of omission rather than commission. The clinically short situation is a marker of skills that we are ready to learn but don't quite have yet.) A man about 60 years of age came for a hearing aid evaluation. He had recently been remarried after spending the previous 5 years as a widower. His new wife was very distressed at his inability to hear and was constantly nagging him to get a hearing aid. He did have an old aid that he had kept in a drawer and wore only occasionally and not very enthusiastically. It was clear from his manner and some of his statements that he was requesting the hearing aid evaluation only at the insistence of his wife, who had not accompanied him to the examination. At that point in my clinical development, I didn't think I had any option but to fulfill the expectations of the client, so I proceeded to test his hearing (he had a steeply sloping audiogram with rather poor speech discrimination) and to try a variety of hearing aids. We found one that was reasonably satisfactory, and I wrote a prescription for the aid (we were not dispensing in those days). My "counseling" consisted of telling him how the aid worked and talking to him about situations in which to use the aid. He never returned for a follow-up visit.

All the time I was testing him and counseling him, I knew I needed to be doing something else. This situation demanded a response other than the traditional approach of audiologist as technician. What I realized somewhat later (3 years, to be exact) was that the wife who was not present also had a hearing-related problem. Because she was also affected by her husband's hearing problem, it was my responsibility to help her by including her in the evaluation. If I could see this case again, I would have stopped the evaluation at the case history stage and suggested that we set up another appointment so that the wife could be present. At the next meeting, having the wife present during the evaluation would have demonstrated to her the limits of his hearing and the limits of amplification for him. We could then have embarked on a discussion of ways to compensate around the home for his reduced acuity. To have included the wife would have been a much more effective clinical strategy than proceeding as I did in treating only the identified patient.

These clinically short situations provide the professional with irritant seeds that can lead to the development of clinical "pearls." I reaffirmed my prior conviction of how important the family was, and the wisdom that evolved from this less-than-satisfactory clinical encounter led me to develop a family-centered nursery program for young children with hearing impairment. I also insisted from that point on that any clients be accompanied by a family member. I think I became a much more effective clinician, which is the usual result of solving a clinically short situation.

My search to become a more effective clinician led me to the literature in family therapy, which I think is incredibly fruitful for our field and is only now beginning to affect the profession of communication disorders. No one person is credited with developing the field of family therapy. Instead, the field seems to have developed spontaneously from the work of several disparate clinicians trained to provide individual therapy. Virginia Satir, Nathan Ackerman, Don Jackson, Salvador Minuchin, Murray Bowen, and Carl Whitaker were forerunners of the current work being done in family therapy (Hoffman, 1981).

At a workshop I attended, Satir told of her introduction to family work. She was a trained psychiatric social worker who was assigned to the back wards of a mental hospital. (I have always wondered about the assignments of new teachers and clinicians to the patients or classes that nobody else wants and that all the experienced professionals consider hopeless. I often thought that these classes and clients needed the most experienced clinicians rather than the neophytes, and the system struck me as absurd. But, as I have reflected on it, perhaps the young clinician does not know that these cases are hopeless and thus gets a better result than the experienced clinician. Clients have a way of responding to clinician expectations.) Satir found that, as her very disturbed patients were getting better, they were earning weekend passes. When they returned on Monday, she found them more disturbed than when they had left on Friday. She realized that working at the identified patient level was not efficient and began insisting that family members attend the counseling sessions. As family members began to interact with the identified patient, Satir found that the whole family was dysfunctional and that the patient's illness played a vital role in maintaining the family homeostasis (Satir, 1967). Very often the identified patient was instrumental in sustaining the parents' marriage by distracting the parents from their marital conflicts. Satir took the whole family in therapy, with excellent results.

Minuchin, Rosman, and Baker (1978) examined families in which children had psychosomatic illnesses. Looking at families of asthmatic, anorectic, and diabetic children who could not maintain appropriate blood sugar levels, they found almost invariably in these families that the marital relationships were in poor shape and that the children's symptoms were a maintaining factor in the families. The "ill" child in each family had been triangulated into the marital conflict, and the symptoms served to keep the family together, although at a huge cost to the child. If patients were to get better, the family homeostasis would be threatened, so everyone within the family was invested in keeping the identified patient "sick." Minuchin and other family therapists now direct their clinical energies at the parental level rather than the child level. This approach has yielded highly successful results (Hoffman, 1981).

The basic notion underlying all family therapy is that the family is a system in which all of the components are interdependent. Every family member affects every other component of the family; for the family therapist, there is no such thing as individual therapy—any time a change occurs in one member of the family, everybody in the family is impacted. Working in individual therapy with an identified patient in a dysfunctional family burdens the individual to become a change agent for the family. This is often too difficult a task for the patient, especially if the patient is a child. Family therapists find it much more efficacious to work at the systems level; in fact, many family therapists refuse to work with individuals.

In our field, we work with families that are under a great deal of stress because they include a person with a communication disorder. These are not necessarily dysfunctional families, only stressed families. Nevertheless, many of the notions developed by family therapists have profound implications for our field, as reflected in our literature.

Egolf, Shames, Johnson, and Kasprisin-Burrell (1972) found that working

with young stutterers within the clinic was not sufficient to effect cures and recommended that clinicians work instead with the parent–child dyad. They wrote,

> If the child adjusts to his environment by stuttering, then the parents must
> have made an equal adjustment in maintaining stuttering—thus the dyad is
> in balance (equilibrium). If treatment changes one member of the dyad, the
> child, by making him fluent, the dyad is forced into disequilibrium. A new
> equilibrium requires changes in both parent and child. (p. 223)

Robertson and Suinn (1968) found a direct correlation between the empathy of
family members and the recovery rate of stroke patients. Edgerly (1975) found
that a program that provided parent education and tutoring yielded significantly
more gains in academic achievement for children having learning disabilities
than a regular curriculum program. He concluded that parents must be directly
involved in a treatment program for it to be successful. Berry (1987) described
techniques and strategies for involving parents in programs for young children
using augmentative and alternative communication systems. She concluded
that the success of an augmentative communication program is dependent in
large part on the attitudes of the family members. Byrne (2000), working with
a school-age hearing-impaired child, compared three conditions of language
learning: parent alone, parent–clinician, and clinician alone. She found that
the least effective condition was taught by the clinician alone and "that across
all instructional methods the parent provided more opportunities than the professional for the child to experience the language target" (p. 217).

The utilization of parents dates back to some of our field's earlier practitioners. Matis (1961) wrote about the need to counsel parents and how it could
be done within a one-clinician setting. In language therapy, the movement
toward pragmatics has brought to the fore the importance of the communicative context, which, for children, is mainly the family. This means that speech
pathologists need to involve themselves with the family. Lund (1986), in a
comprehensive article on family and language intervention, commented,

> In the family context the child learns a style of relating as well as vocabulary
> and grammar that will be carried into all subsequent communication situa-
> tions. We want to highlight and learn from those aspects of the family's in-
> teraction that promote effective communication and work with the family to
> decrease those aspects that seem to impede communication. (p. 417)

Superior and Leichook (1986) argued cogently for involving the parents in
a school-based language intervention program. They felt that increased knowledge by the parents about the language disorder leads to more acceptance and

sensitivity to the restrictions that their children may encounter, and that including the parents leads to greater carryover into the home environment and to preventive education. If the parents can learn to become strong language models who will facilitate growth in the child's language, the development of further disorders will be prevented. The authors developed a parent-consultation model to be implemented in a public school setting. Girolametta, Greenberg, and Manolson (1986) described a parent program for developing parents' dialogue skills with their children. Andrews (1986), a trained family therapist who worked in conjunction with a speech pathologist, described techniques for treating language disorders within a family-based approach. From their work with families of children with cochlear implants, DesJardin, Eisenberg, and Hodapp (2006) concluded,

> Early intervention programs that capitalize on parents' sense of knowledge and competence will empower parents as they support their child's development. Parental involvement and self efficacy are critical aspects to consider as professionals support language learning in families of young children with cochlear implants. (p. 186)

The literature contains little information about the families of catastrophically ill adults, and few programs seem to be available. Emerson (1980), after a careful review of the literature on families of individuals with aphasia, concluded that "involving the family in rehabilitation is more often stressed in theory than actually practiced" (p. 23). He provided a group experience for the spouses of aphasic patients and found that after group therapy, the spouses showed gains in self-esteem and were less depressed compared with a control group that did not undergo group therapy. Within the spouse group, opportunity was provided for the exploration and confirmation of feelings. Bardach (1969), in conjunction with a speech pathologist, conducted group sessions with wives of patients with aphasia. She found that these group sessions were immensely helpful, and she, like almost everyone who has written in the field, laments the lack of widespread support programs for families. M. Webster (1982), an adult who suffered a cerebrovascular accident, commented, "Had someone been able to counsel with my family about what to expect from me, their lives would have been much easier" (p. 235).

Malone (1969) interviewed the families of 20 adults with aphasia. He found that the aphasia created severe stress for the family, which in turn aggravated the condition of the patient. Probably the most pervasive change noted was the role reversal: Wives who had been taken care of by their husbands were suddenly themselves caretakers; husbands who had never assumed any domestic responsibility were now required to do housework in addition to continuing as the breadwinners; children were now required to take care of parents. Families were further stressed by financial problems, health problems, and severe alterations to their social lives. Not surprisingly, these changes generated feelings of guilt and anger. The guilt arose from a feeling that the aphasia was a punishment for a wrong done; the anger was caused by the loss of control.

Kommers and Sullivan (1979) gathered questionnaire data from the wives of laryngectomized men. They found that the families had problems with health, communication, finances, and occupation. More than 50% of the younger wives reported marital changes after the laryngectomy. This study did not provide any interview material, but I think it is safe to assume that many of the same difficulties that affected the families of adults with aphasia (Malone, 1969) would be shown to affect the families of laryngectomized patients.

Alpiner (1978) also found little in the literature about the families of adults with acquired hearing loss. He recommended that the audiologist see the family initially without the hearing-impaired member to help them understand the hearing loss. He then suggested that, if possible, family members attend therapy sessions.

Fleming (1972) proposed essentially a family counseling approach with hard-of-hearing adults. After a comprehensive audiologic workup, the person with hearing impairment is urged to attend group sessions accompanied by a family member. At these sessions, the families work out strategies for coping with the hearing impairment. They also have an opportunity to ventilate and share their feelings. For example, in one session I attended, a wife was complaining bitterly about being a "hearing-ear dog" for her husband; she was tired of having to answer the phone, explain the punch lines of jokes, and translate television programs. She received confirmation of her feelings from the other spouses in the group, and she and her husband were able to devise, with the help of the audiologist present, some techniques to increase his adaptation to the hearing loss. The couple was able to obtain amplifiers for the phone and the television; they were also able to work out some living strategies that would minimize his dependency. In addition, the cathartic experience within the group setting enabled the couple to work constructively on the problem once the interfering feelings had been discharged.

I think the field of communication disorders is gradually coming to realize the efficacy of working at the family level. Federal legislation, such as the Education of the Handicapped Act Amendments of 1986 (P.L. 99-457), mandates our involvement at the family level. I think also that as we mature as a profession and throw off our technician shackles, we are recognizing the need to work at a family level. To do this successfully, we need to understand how the family system functions and the various roles that significant family members play.

Components of the Family

Spouses

All marriages involve a contract (Sager, 1978). The contract comprises a set of expectations and promises that may or may not be shared with the spouse. More often than not, the contract is implied. There are three levels of contracts: (a) conscious and verbalized, (b) conscious and not verbalized, and (c) unconscious. The marital partners enter their relationship with separate contractual expectations and then work toward developing a single joint marital contract. The early conflicts that couples have are usually part of a healthy process of forging the joint contract.

A major source of marital conflict occurs when there is contractual disappointment. Despite the marriage vow "in sickness and in health," one never really expects to or is prepared to deal with severe long-term disability in a spouse. Each marriage partner is usually psychologically protected against thinking about or planning for spousal disability by the myth of invulnerability that we all use to assuage our anxiety over dealing with the existential issues. Each spouse's dream of what marriage and life will be like does not include a spousal disability. When a spouse becomes disabled by, for example, a stroke or severe hearing loss, the contract is violated. Spouses are usually enormously angry and feel somehow cheated. They are grief-stricken at the loss of their dream; they sometimes feel guilty that they may have done something to cause the disability. They recognize their vulnerability and are frightened and anxious about the future. Above all else, spouses feel an overwhelming loneliness due to the loss of a marital partner with whom they planned to share their life and in whom they confided. One man in a disability group I was facilitating lamented, "I have lost my best friend."

Many spouses have nobody with whom to share the burden of caring for the spouse who is disabled. At the time of diagnosis or early signs of disease, the crisis usually pulls a family together. Short-term difficulties cause people in the family to set aside their personal agendas and rise above individual problems to help one another; the immediate crisis has a way of bringing out the best in most people. After the initial crisis, when family members realize the person is permanently disabled and the problem turns out to be a long-term, chronic disability, the angers and resentments emerge and the disappointments become a divisive factor in many families. The well spouse is usually left "holding the bag." The loneliness is acute. Many marriages founder because of the disability of a spouse (or the illness in a child), but many others are strengthened by the crisis.

The marital subsystem within the family is generally a delicately balanced system that is always seeking equilibrium. In addition to being a contract, a marriage is a balancing act. Partners generally marry someone who has qualities that they admire and feel are lacking in themselves; for example, people with a cognitive bent are often attracted to mates who deal with the world from an intuitive, feeling stance. This is what sociologists call "marrying complementary," and within the family unit, very often there is a congruence that is absent in any one member of the marital pair. Thus, if one person is outgoing, the other is inhibited; if he is a talker, she is a listener; if he is an accumulator, she is a thrower-outer. This congruence is useful to the family during times of crisis; when one spouse is emotionally and cognitively devastated, the other is able to keep the family afloat by dealing with all the information that needs to be processed. The equilibrium is maintained almost unconsciously; if one spouse is "down" on the emotional seesaw, the other has to be "up." I remember a wife complaining that her husband never seemed to grieve over their child's deafness; he was always cheering her up, as she was often a "basket case." It wasn't until a year later that he suddenly broke down and cried. It was no accident that his letting go coincided with his wife's feeling good about her ability to cope; this now gave him permission to grieve. Unfortunately, in some families, one spouse will get locked into the "up" role and never have any space or permission to grieve. When partners are locked into their emotional and physical roles, there invariably is a great deal of marital stress, because there is a restriction on each individual's ability to grow. In a comprehensive article on couples in which one partner has a neurological disability, Ventimiglia (1986) listed those factors that would lead to the preservation of the relationship. Among them are the following:

1. If the disability is mild

2. If there is an abundance of resources

3. If the marital contract is renegotiated

4. If tolerable substitutions are made for lost activities

5. If some sense is made of the tragedy

6. If the well spouse is prone to nurturance (men are more likely to leave a disability marriage than women)

He commented that in many cases, "divorce becomes a matter of survival, not the pursuit of happiness" (p. 125).

In my experience working with groups of healthy spouses of individuals with chronic illness, I have found that the families that grow and prosper through the adversity of the disability are the older, longer married couples whose companionship has been tested over time. The others that succeed are the newly married couples who enter the marriage knowing about the disability and have openly and honestly made their choice. No matter how well prepared people may think they are for marriage to someone with a disability, they really cannot know how they will react until they experience it. The pain—of today and the rest of one's life—ultimately wears down a well spouse. Caring for someone on a short-term basis or only in a peripheral capacity is relatively easy; one can be loving and giving if he or she can plan to return to a normal life in a short while.

The couples most at risk are those who have been married only a few years and have not been subjected to enough external stress to strengthen them, or those who have not yet established openness in their marital communication. These marriages are much more likely to crumble under the added weight of a disability.

Having a spouse with a chronic disability does not necessarily lead to divorce or estrangement. The disability causes marital stress by altering the marriage contract and violating expectations, thus exposing weakness that might otherwise be papered over. With some marriages, the exposed cracks are so deep that the foundation crumbles. In other marriages, the stress caused by the disability is an occasion for working and strengthening the marital bond and cementing the cracks so that a stronger foundation can be put in place.

The professional in communication disorders needs to direct considerable clinical attention to the well spouse. This time is well spent and will have an enormous long-term impact on the client. By supporting and educating the spouse, the professional can help create a home that is facilitative for the client. Unfortunately, this does not happen often enough. In a spousal group I was facilitating, one wife said, "I have had multiple sclerosis for 17 years, only nobody knows it." Another spouse said, "In this concert I am always playing second violin." Programmatically, we need to look at these "second fiddles."

We need to redirect our professional energies toward making the well spouse our first priority; if we take good care of the spouse, the identified patient has a much better chance of doing well. We need to include the spouse in all diagnostic workups as well as in therapy with the client. Rollins (1988) described the reactions of spouses of individuals with aphasia and the implications for counseling; he recommended actively involving the spouses in therapy and diagnosis. Some spouses are so locked in denial and anger that it seems we cannot reach them. We need to listen to and support them as we work to enhance their self-esteem. They may then give up the denial; as we listen and avoid judgment, they may have a chance to ventilate their anger.

Above all else, we must provide for the spouses a support group in which some of their loneliness can be abated. Having worked intensively with spousal groups, I have become ever more certain of the value of a support group to provide a healing environment.

In the early sessions of a well-spouse group, there is an immense sense of relief and a rush of long-pent-up emotions emerging like a dam bursting. It is almost palpable. Finally, there is a venue where well spouses can find mutual understanding and the members can be accepted as they talk about their problems without feeling guilty or whining. After the first few sessions, which are mainly cathartic, the group usually begins sharing information as it moves from an emotion-centered focus to a problem-centered focus. Members often leave feeling supported; they have established a network of friends that can relieve the crushing loneliness of living with a chronically ill person.

Parents

According to Minuchin (1974), modern parenting is essentially an impossible task. He felt, and I agree wholeheartedly, that "parenting is an extremely difficult task that no one performs to his entire satisfaction and no one goes through the process unscathed" (p. 83). There is always conflict within the parental task. Parents cannot protect and guide a child without recourse, at times, to being controlling and restrictive. On the other hand, children cannot grow without testing the limits imposed by their parents, thus being seen by their parents as rejecting and hostile. Parents often are in conflict not only with their children, but with themselves as to whether they are fulfilling their nurturing function or their controlling–guiding function. The chronic dilemma of all parents is determining in a given situation how much control they should maintain and how much freedom they should give to their children. The parents' job is to gradually cede control to the child, but the timing of the release of control is very difficult to determine. If parents cede control too quickly, the child will have negative experiences that can lead to feelings of incompetency. If the parents hold on too long, the child will receive the message that he or she is incompetent to deal with the world. Both premature and delayed release of control generally have the same result: a fearful, low-risk child. There is a relatively small margin of control that the parent has to work with; a disability in the child limits the margins even further.

According to Satir (1967), "The parents are the axis around which all other family relationships are formed; the mates are the architects of the family" (p. 63). The marital relationship affects the parenting. When parents are close and supportive of each other, they are better able to fulfill their parental responsibilities. When parents are not close emotionally, very often the child gets "triangulated" into the marriage. As discussed earlier, the child may develop psychosomatic symptoms in order to salvage the parental marriage. Triangulation often occurs when the child is born with a disability.

According to Mendelsohn and Rozek (1983), the

> intrinsic characteristics of the deafness and the caretaking process lend themselves to the child being easily triangulated into the anxious or conflictual areas in the family life; the disability puts the child into focus more easily because of the need for more attention and care. (p. 39)

Pedersen (1976) examined families with a child with a disability and found that when there was an emotionally distant husband, there was an emotionally distant mother. The mother's ability to parent well was a function in large part of the satisfaction she obtained in her marriage. Gallagher, Cross, and Scharfman (1981) identified the characteristics of parents who were judged by professionals to have made a successful adjustment to the birth of a child with a disability. The data suggested that the major sources of strength were the parents' personal qualities and the quality of the husband–wife relationship.

The triangle consisting of the parents and the child is most apparent in preschool programs, where it is not uncommon to find a distant father. Programs usually try to strengthen the father–child bond by seducing the father into involvement with the program. A conference of educators of individuals with hearing impairment devoted an entire session to involving fathers in home intervention (SKI-HI, 1985). Among the suggestions developed were that the professional make an effort to establish rapport with the father early, take time to write or leave notes for him, call him at work, give him assignments, and always reinforce him for his work with the child. I think these strategies will work nicely in families in which the father is timid about involving himself with his child. This is especially true with first-time fathers of very young children. It must be kept in mind, however, that system theory would predict that when the father–child relationship is altered, the mother–child relationship and the husband–wife relationship will be altered as well. One leg of the triangle cannot change without affecting the other parts.

Very often, however, attempts to attract the father fail completely or succeed only momentarily before the father resumes his distant behavior. Invariably, the professional starts searching for another gimmick to attract the father or enters into a subtle coalition with the mother that only further excludes and alienates the father. This is always a mistake.

If we wish to, we can affect the father–child relationship by working with the mother–child dyad or the husband–wife relationship. In families with distant fathers, mothers frequently are very closely bonded to their children, sometimes to the point that they do not want the father present at all, despite their protestations to the contrary. Many of these mothers have unresolved feelings of guilt, and they feel that repairing the damage is their responsibility. Also, for many mothers, the child with a disability becomes the means for realizing their self-worth; they discover the joy of working with their child and gain confidence in their ability to do the job well. The child gives direction and meaning to their lives. Consequently, they do not want the fathers to "mess up" their work. Very often a father is insecure and incompetent in doing what needs to be done, and the mother would rather do it herself. She either consciously or unconsciously excludes or intimidates him. Very often the presence of a child with a disability triggers a spiral into marital discord. When the mother becomes overinvolved with the child, little energy is left for the marriage. When the father is getting little satisfaction within the marriage, he will seek involvement somewhere else—usually work. As he becomes more involved in work, she becomes more involved in parenting, which leaves him to become further involved in work, and so it goes until there is little or no energy left for the marriage.

Some wives need to have a club to wield over their husbands. The father's physical and emotional distance from the child with a disability often becomes the weapon. The mother frequently gets emotional support from other family members and sometimes from professionals against the "bad" father by "doing it" alone. It is always poor case management for the speech pathologist or audiologist to enter into an alliance with the mother against the father. If we examined the parents' marriage closely, we would invariably find a great deal of conflict; the fight over the child is usually only one of many long-simmering disputes.

Another thing we have to bear in mind is that some families can be quite successful with a clinically distant father. Because families work in many different ways, professionals need to respect the individual family's coping strategy as long as the family remains functional. A coping strategy that requires an overinvolved mother may be necessary if the family is to turn out a successfully functioning child who has a disability. This solution will work if the mother feels that she is supported and that her burden is shared with the family; the father who assumes some of the mother's chores at home while she is at the child's school is emotionally supportive of her and can be a very effective father who never appears at the clinic. There may be no need for him to enter the clinic or to be involved directly with his child's therapy. Sometimes there is much truth in the statement that the best thing a father can do for his children is to love his wife.

Women professionals who are at a different stage of social consciousness than the children's mothers often judge a family as deficient if it is run with traditional sex-role stereotypes. These families can be, and very often are, quite successful and functional as long as everyone is content with his or her roles. The family must always be accepted for what it *is* rather than for what the professional feels it *should be*. We must always have sensitivity to the multicultural differences among families and never impose our values on the families we are working with. Matkin (1998) repeatedly makes the case for professionals being culturally sensitive to the families' values in working with the families of deaf children.

In the Emerson College program, we make no special efforts to coax fathers to attend, although they are always very welcome. We offer evening meetings for fathers if the parents wish, or we have a Saturday nursery each semester to accommodate working parents. These are offered only if the parents so request. I have worked with many families in the program without ever meeting the fathers or having only limited contact. In addition, many single-parent families are successful in the program.

The emotions involved in having a child with a disability are very intense. Featherstone (1980) noted that a child's disability strains the marriage by evoking such strong emotions in both parents that it becomes "a fertile source of conflict and disrupts the organization of the family on a long-term basis. The disabled child is always a symbol of a shared failure" (p. 172). Gath (1977) studied each of 30 families with a child with Down syndrome for 5 years after the birth of the child, as well as a carefully controlled group of 30 families with nondisabled children. At the end of the 5-year period, she found that nine of the families with a child with Down syndrome experienced severe marital discord, whereas none of the control families reported severe difficulties.

Anger is potentially the most destructive emotion in the marriage. The parents usually have no satisfactory outlet for anger. Many do not even recognize anger, and others repress it, and then it emerges as depression. In families where the expression of anger is not sanctioned, anger is often displaced; the parents may argue about the quality of the cooking or the whiteness of the laundry. In the early stages of diagnosis and therapy, the parents' fights are seldom over what actually angers them. Fear, the loss of control, and the impotence they feel in the face of their child's disability fuel many a fight. Much of the anger is also displaced onto the professionals.

Guilt is also potentially destructive to a marriage if it is not recognized and dealt with effectively. Guilt is usually felt by both parents, although mothers—because they carried the child during the pregnancy—seem to carry a heavier freight of it. Because guilt is such an uncomfortable feeling, the parents try to push it off on each other. Thus begins the search through their family trees to find some defective relative, preferably on the other spouse's side of the family; in combination with rage, guilt can be a formidable divisive force. The anger and blaming that parents can fall into has split many a marriage.

With guilt often comes the "superdedicated" parent who is committed to "making it up" to the child with a disability, usually at the expense of the rest of the family. Less attention is paid to the husband–wife relationship and to the nondisabled siblings. The parent often ignores his or her own needs and becomes one-dimensional—almost monomaniacal. The child's disability becomes the dominating force in the family to the exclusion and resentment of everyone else. If allowed to, the child with a disability can consume an inordinate amount of energy and radically alter the family structure.

In most families, the parents do not synchronize their feelings or are unwilling to share their feelings because they feel they would be imposing. For example, a mother in a parent group spoke about not wanting to tell her husband her fears and anxieties because that just "sets him off." She kept stating, "We aren't very good for each other because we pull each other down." It is also difficult to deal with one parent who is heavily in denial while the other is overtly deeply distressed. Both parents feel that they lack support from the other, and each feels that the spouse does not understand what is occurring.

Frequently, a spouse finds it difficult to listen to and respond to the other's pain. This seems especially true of husbands. Men frequently assign themselves the role of family protector; when a member of the family is in pain about which the man can do nothing, he feels responsible and impotent. This emotion often triggers a denial reaction. Many men refuse to talk about feelings because to do so undermines their own denial mechanism. They then try to distract their wives from pain in order to make the wives feel better, usually with disastrous results. (In actuality, they are trying to make themselves feel better, and this needs to be pointed out.) The inability or unwillingness of parents to talk about their feelings can be divisive. The professional needs to help the parents resolve the issue of managing each other's grief. The professional needs to be a person with whom parents can talk and cry without having their feelings invalidated. Often it is desirable to bring both parents together to discuss the dynamics of their relationship as it is affected by grief. It is often necessary to try to release the husband from the protector role in order to allow him to grieve and then leave space in their relationship for the wife's grief.

Yalom (1989) said the following about working with grieving parents:

> Therapy has much to offer grieving parents. Couples' treatment may illuminate the source of marital tension and help each partner to recognize and respect the other's mode of grief. Individual therapy may help to alter dysfunctional mourning. Wary though I am always of generalizations, in this instance male-female stereotypes also hold true. Many women need to move past the repetitive expression of their loss and to plunge back into engagement with the living, with projects, with all the things that may supply meaning for their own lives. Men usually must be taught to experience and share (rather than to suppress and evade) their sadness. (p. 142)

Many changes in the family structure occur when a child with a disability is introduced. The husband–wife relationship is altered radically; wives may have to postpone their careers even further; and economic hardships can occur. Plans are formulated based on the availability of schooling, and difficult family choices have to be made. Families often need a place to talk about these changes and their stresses. In many programs, the parent education becomes, in fact, mother education. Very often the mother, by virtue of being actively involved in the educational program, possesses more information and is in a better position to make decisions regarding the child's welfare than is the father. In some families that have a very set sex-role orientation, the changing role of the wife can be a threat to marital stability. Over the 40-year history of the Emerson College program, we have seen marriages founder. I am not sure that the number of failed marriages in this population is any greater than the national statistic on divorce, which is alarming, but clearly the child with a disability does add more stress to the marriage. I do not consider divorce a failure. Very often it is a solution, albeit painful, to a difficult situation. I think children are better off in a divorced family than in one in which there is no communication or love between the parents.

In the Emerson College program, families are an important element. In addition to attending the support group once a week (usually the mother attends, but not always), parents are required to participate with their child in the nursery at least one morning a week. The nursery is staffed by an early childhood professional instead of a teacher of the deaf. (The Emerson College program is for children with hearing loss, but the discerning reader can see that this format is appropriate for children with other disabilities as well.) I think it is very important that we pay attention to the child's developmental needs first and then the special needs related to the hearing loss. To this end we always include in the nursery a hearing child, not to stimulate language, but to remind us all of the developmental issues of a 2-year-old. One chronic problem that parents have is trying to distinguish between the behavior that is due to the hearing loss and the behavior that is due to developmental issues. One fantasy that parents verbalize is, "If I could just speak to my child, all of the problems would clear up." They realize this is a fantasy when they watch staff try to deal with the hearing child. The mother of the hearing child sometimes participates in the parent group, and the mothers of the deaf children usually realize that she is having as many management problems as they are. (Perhaps the deafest creature on the face of the earth is a 2-year-old, with or without a hearing loss.)

Usually eight children between the ages of 18 months and 3 years are in the nursery with the nursery school teacher and several graduate students from a speech pathology program. The nursery is equipped with a large one-way mirror through which parents observe their children. The children have individual speech–language therapy each day in adjoining therapy rooms, also equipped with one-way mirrors for parental observation. As the program progresses (we operate on an academic calendar from September to June), the parents begin to take over the program. Instead of watching, they take turns working with the children in the nursery and in therapy, while staff watches. By springtime, it is often hard to tell by casual observation who are staff members and who are parents. At all points we seek to empower parents.

With the advent of newborn screening, infants as young as 3 months of age are entering our program. In fact, now we rarely start working with a family when the child is toddler age. The infant program provides one-on-one therapy with a speech–language pathologist and also encourages parents to participate in the support group. In some years, when we have had a sufficient number of infants, we have held a special group for the parents of infants. The preference now is to mix the groups, as there is a great deal of value in the "cross-generational" experiences of parents of toddlers and parents of infants. Parents a little further along the habilitation path can be immensely helpful to those parents just beginning their journey. It is also beneficial for the parents with older children to see how far they have come, and for parents of infants to get a sense of validation and hope that the intense pain they now feel will pass.

Over the years, our definition of *parent* has evolved as more mothers have gone to work outside the home. We enroll any family in the program as long as a primary caregiver is present. We have worked on occasion with aunts, grandparents, and babysitters. We will not enroll any child without an accompanying caregiver. We feel it is presumptuous to think that by working 5 or 6 hours a week with only the child, we can effect massive changes; however, by spending that time with the adults, we can impact the child all the time by altering the home environment. It is much more efficacious to work this way.

Fathers seldom receive or solicit emotional support. Almost all support seems to be directed toward the mothers. Yet many fathers do need to be listened to and need to be able to talk about their feelings—a fact they may not even realize. Programs need to provide opportunities for the fathers to participate without stressing the marital contract. Fathers can be invited, and if they do not attend, that needs to be accepted as well.

Crowley, Keane, and Needham (1982) held a series of bimonthly evening meetings with fathers of children enrolled in a school for the deaf. During the first year, they offered a rather structured content-based program; they then moved into an unstructured group discussion that encouraged more self-disclosure and feelings. Both fathers and staff concluded that the program was very successful. I suspect that the more structured, content-based program may be a good entry point for most fathers. Most men seem to find it difficult to talk about feelings, and if some trust and cohesion can develop in the group while dealing with structured content, it may be easier for the men to move subsequently into affect areas.

In the Emerson College program, we have held nursery on a Saturday morning at least once each semester so that fathers could attend. We have had evening group meetings with fathers only, and we have had husband-and-wife groups. In the latter groups, it was difficult to get much openness, as each parent did not want to reveal very much for fear of angering his or her spouse. One semester we held a group in which half the men and half the women attended without their spouses. We held a second meeting with the other halves; this group was a great deal more open, and there was a strong confidentiality norm.

We have also experimented with intensive weekend experiences without the children. Staff and parents spend 2 days together in a resort setting. Time is set aside for reflection and recreation as well as group meetings. Within this setting, I have used a fishbowl design where one group sits in the center and the rest of the group is silent and on the periphery. The fathers, for example, may talk about how they are affected by their children's deafness while the mothers listen. Then the mothers talk while the fathers listen. At the end of the session, everybody processes the experience. I always try to conclude an intense husband–wife encounter with the couples going off to a corner and taking turns telling each other what they appreciate about the other person. Other sessions are devoted to large-group discussion. The fishbowl format, in conjunction with the intensive weekend experience, has given us very cohesive parent groups. There has been greater father participation and involvement in all aspects of the program when we have been able to utilize the intensive weekend. (Unfortunately, costs have precluded our using this strategy for the past several years.) I have also worked with programs for deaf children that include a learning vacation for the families. I find that there is the same intensity of experience in these groups as there is in the clinic-based programs, and they are among the most satisfying that I do, albeit on a very short-term basis.

My experience suggests that although the presence of a child with a disability in the family creates stress, there are also significant positives for many families that have a child with a disability. The stress can be an occasion for growth. Kazak and Marvin (1984) found that in 56 families in which a child had spinal bifida, a significant portion of the parents reported that their marriage was strengthened as a result of the child. Likewise, a mother of a 5-year-old deaf child said,

> I really grew to appreciate my husband these last few years. He has really risen to the occasion. He has gone with me to all important meetings and he takes over a great deal of the day-to-day responsibility from me. I never knew he cared so deeply for me and my child until this happened.

The professional, by working sensitively, can help the family achieve a positive outcome from the experience of having a child with a disability. I think a major key to working with the parents is to give them permission to take care of themselves first. A valuable metaphor for me has been the instructions I receive from the flight attendant whenever I fly. He or she tells me that if an oxygen mask should be needed and I am traveling with a child, I should put a mask on my face first and then take care of the child. This makes powerful sense to me because in order to give, I have to be getting from someplace, and if I go under there is nobody to take care of the child. If I am to take good care of somebody else, I have to start by taking good care of myself. Parents often don't see this simple truth; they tend to give, give, and give until they are burnt out and resentful. If they do something for themselves, they usually feel very guilty. One thing I have learned in the past 40 years is that happy parents turn out well-functioning children. If they can take some time for themselves and for strengthening their marriages, they will be better parents. The counseling program needs to provide an avenue for the parents to find their happiness. Each time I work with a parent group, I am struck anew by how much growth and joy can emerge from so much pain and suffering.

The Children of Parents With Disability

The need to view one's parents as strong, intelligent, and very competent is a childhood illusion that is difficult to alter at any age. It is hard to know when childhood ends; we have no real markers. My brother has commented that the time he was most frightened while growing up was when he talked about a family problem and our parents actually listened to him.

Adolescents are normally granted a moratorium or postponement period during which the identity of childhood gradually merges with that of adulthood. Eventually the adolescent must give up this moratorium to assume adult responsibility. Adolescence is a cultural and social event. The biology is clear: One moment the person is a child and the next minute he or she is capable of having children. Adolescence is a luxury that society can afford only when it is affluent. In marginal societies, the adolescent joins the workforce in order to contribute to the society as early as possible, and in poor families in an affluent society, the adolescent is often called on to assume adult responsibilities sooner than their more well-off counterparts. My father, for example, the son of immigrant parents, left school after eighth grade to join the workforce and become an important contributor to the family. He never had an adolescence and could not cope very well with mine (I don't know many parents who can); we had a stormy relationship until shortly before his death.

Probably the best indication of when someone has arrived at adulthood is the willingness to see one's parents as fellow adults struggling with the very human problems of making the most of their lives. There is a very predictable life crisis of adulthood that occurs when we realize that we are more capable than our parents. This is not the adolescent experience that Mark Twain described when he quipped, "When I was 15, I thought my father was the stupidest person alive. At 19 I was surprised at how much he had learned in four short years."

There does come a crisis point for all of us, usually in our adulthood, when we realize we actually do know more than our parents. There is a role reversal that occurs, and we then begin to parent our parents. This realization usually leaves us feeling frightened and alone because we often experience our existential aloneness and recognize that there is nobody left to protect us. For most of us, the realization of our dominion over our parents usually occurs over time, fueled by many small incidents that reflect our parents' increasing incompetence.

For adolescent children of parents with a disability, the moratorium phase is shortened or sometimes becomes even nonexistent as these children become "parentified" and are forced to assume adult responsibilities much sooner than their peers. For these children, the normal crisis of adulthood is accelerated. They have to deal with parental incompetence at a much earlier age than they might be ready for developmentally. This can be quite frightening to self-absorbed adolescents, who ordinarily see parents as unwanted intrusions on their autonomy or merely as providers for their sustenance, but rarely as people.

To have to suddenly look at your father as someone who can no longer be a provider, but rather as a person who is hurting and fearful and who may now be dependent on you, is quite frightening.

There is very little information in the literature about how children of parents with disability fare. Roy (1990), in a review of the literature of children of adults with a disability, concluded, "How much attention should the clinician pay to the children of chronically ill parents? Common sense suggests a great deal but research evidence remains equivocal" (p. 120). In my experience interviewing families and working with them professionally, I have found that the children can go either of two ways: They become parentified early and lose their adolescence while becoming responsible young adults, or they act out their fears and perceived lack of attention by getting into trouble. Children can survive and grow under adverse conditions; what they cannot sustain is indifference, and as long as they feel cared for by the parents, they will respond and grow. The problem is whether or not the parents have any energy left to deal with their children's problems while they are wrestling with the formidable problems engendered by their own disability.

We do know that children are sensitive barometers of family stress. All writers on the subject agree that life is stressful for the child of a parent with a disability, but the stress can work either way; it can be a maturing factor and produce a very responsible child, or it can lead to neglect and become a springboard for delinquent behavior. It seems to me that the children's success or lack of it is almost always a function of how well the parents are coping with the disease process. When the parents are able to get the disease in perspective, so that it is no longer dominating their every waking thought and consuming their psychic and physical energy, then they can devote time to their children. Until this happens, the children (especially in the early stages of diagnosis) are pretty much on their own. If there was strength in the family to begin with, then the child can survive and even flourish. In weaker family systems, the children and family itself may not be able to survive without considerable scarring.

The effect of parental chronic illness on the adult child who has left the family is also variable depending in large part on that child's designated role in the family and how close both physically and emotionally that child is to the parent. Some children within the family structure become designated early as caretakers. This role usually devolves onto the oldest female (see sibling section). I have encountered families in which the caretaker was a son, but these have been relatively rare. Most of the research on the adult child of disability has been with Alzheimer's patients. Because the patient is mentally incompetent, researchers are forced to utilize the family.

Dementia, in particular, is an illness striking the patient at the very core of his or her humanness, altering the hallmarks of personality and intelligence.

The worm of the disease burrows deeply within and destroys a person's substance, leaving only the empty husk of the person for others to view. The body remains the same, at least in the early stages, but the mind and personhood, as family members remember it, are gone. There is a psychological death long before physical death, and there are no rituals to help the family through the mourning. It is a never-ending struggle for family members of dementia patients to try to keep fresh the memory of what used to be while dealing with the present reality, which bears no resemblance, in the ways that matter, to the person they knew.

One adult child of a parent with Alzheimer's disease had this to say:

> The crazy thing is that someone has really died two years ago, in essence, yet their actual death is still a horrible process. I don't know what you hang on to. You hang on to something. The difficulty is then of getting that memory of the last stages out of your mind. The impressions are so strong. That's not what you want to remember about them. It's hard to bring them back the way they were. It takes a long time when you remember them, not to remember them the way they were at the end. It happens eventually; it takes time.

Families must always struggle with the decision to institutionalize the parent with dementia: There is invariably guilt that they are failing in their responsibilities, and for many families the decision to institutionalize is an economic one. At $4,000+ a month, most families cannot afford to keep a family member in a nursing home for long, so they attempt to do it themselves, usually at horrendous cost to the health and welfare of the caregiver. The laws are such that families must reduce themselves to a poverty status before they can begin to "afford" a nursing home, and when faced with the twin prospects of poverty or exhaustion, most families opt for exhaustion. The literature is replete with instances where the able-bodied spouse of someone with dementia needed psychiatric care and hospitalization. Depressed and exhausted are the two most frequent descriptors of the caretakers (Baumgarten et al., 1990).

The decision to institutionalize is very complex, involving a host of variables. Among them are the amount of family strain, family finances, support structure of the family, and health of the primary caretaker (Rabins, 1984).

In any event, the family, especially the adult children, must be able to somehow reconstitute their lives after the death of the parent. Nuland (1994) described the problem well:

> It often seems as though the families of Alzheimer's patients are sidetracked from the broad sunlit avenues of ongoing life, remaining trapped for years in its own excruciating cul-de-sac. The only rescue comes with the death of a

person they love. And even then, the memories and the dreadful toll drag on and from these the release can only be partial. A life that has been lived and a shared sense of happiness and accomplishments are ever after seen through the smudged glass of its last few years. For the survivors, the concourse of existence has forever become less bright and less direct. (p. 105)

Perhaps the ultimate act of childhood is the burying of one's parents; for the children of parents with a disability, it is not always clear when the death takes place. What is clear is that the children are called upon to become compassionate, caring adults at an early age, and this is something that many of these children seem to accomplish very well.

Grandparents

At this point in time, there is very little published research about grandparents. Although grandparents often play a very important role in the families that we encounter, they appear to be a badly underresearched, underutilized resource to the family and to the professionals.

The grandparents are present in every family, whether or not they are actively involved. We always carry our family of origin with us into our new nuclear family. Our notions of what constitutes marriage and parenthood stem from our childhood experiences when we observed and assessed our parents' marriage and their parenting. We carry that image with us when we start our new family, either by imitating our parents or by being determined to be different. In either case, we are heavily influenced by them. Only with time and thought do we begin to find our way into marital and parental roles based on our own direct experiences. Some of the change comes about in the initial phases of family formation due to the stress of melding the spouses' disparate personal paradigms into the new family paradigm. Our ideas of what is appropriate and normal stem from our experience in our families of origin and reflect the values of our grandparents.

Grandparenthood is the ultimate developmental phase of parenthood. It is being able to parent without having the responsibility. Probably the one place that the child can have unconditional love is with the grandparents. Parents, because of their civilizing–instructing function, are often in conflict with their children. Grandparents generally have a more loving and accepting relationship with the child. I always knew that if the police were on my tail, my grandmother would take me in. My parents would also take me in, but they would believe the police. My grandmother would always believe me. A cynic has commented that grandparents and grandchildren are natural allies because they both have the same enemy; it is a rare person who has a bad relationship with his or her grandparent.

Unfortunately, the grandparent seems to be rapidly disappearing as an involved member of the family. Based on their interviews of 300 grandparents and grandchildren, Kornhaber and Woodward (1985) reported that only 15% of the families included an actively involved grandparent. The majority (70%) of grandparents were intermittently involved and 15% were not involved at all. The authors of the study felt that a new social contract was in effect that allowed the parents to define the grandparents' role, and the new role diminished grandparent involvement. (I think that the increased affluence that has enabled grandparents to live independently and at a distance from their children also contributes to this diminishing involvement. Extended families used to be a necessity because grandparents could no longer support themselves after retiring; Social Security has changed this.)

Based on their in-depth interviews of the children and the grandparents, Kornhaber and Woodward (1985) found that families benefited from closely connected grandparents. The grandparents functioned as mentors, caretakers, and mediators between the child and the parents; as sex-role models; and as family historians. The results of this study suggested no negative effects of grandparent involvement. A different picture might have emerged if the authors had interviewed the parents, because grandparents can and frequently do introduce stress in the home.

Harris, Handiman, and Palmer (1985) used a questionnaire to interview the parents and grandparents of 19 children with autism. They found that the grandparents had a consistently less pessimistic view of the child's limitations than did the parents. They also noted that grandparents tended to deny the child's disability long after it had been accepted by the parents. Lowe (1989) adapted Harris et al.'s questionnaire for grandparents of 39 deaf children. She found similar results, with the grandparents consistently more optimistic and more locked in denial than the parents.

These studies validate my own clinical observations that grandparents generally lag behind the parents in accepting a child's disability. It is very difficult for the grandparents to deal with the pain of having a grandchild with a disability in conjunction with seeing the pain their own child is experiencing. For the grandparents, it is a double hurt, at a time in life when they are least prepared to cope with emotional emergencies. The grandparents, like most nonprofessionals, lack information and knowledge about the child's disorder. Consequently, their own children frequently know far more than they do, and a role reversal suddenly occurs. The parents, through their professional contacts and by virtue of living with the problem on a daily basis, generally move through the grief stages much faster than the grandparents can. When we are hurting, we generally want and need support from our own parents. The parents of the child with a disability, when they seek support from their own parents, often find it is not there. Instead, the grandparents are seeking information and support from their own children. The parents are then in a role reversal where they are forced to parent their own parents. They often feel cheated and deeply resentful of this reversal because they themselves want badly to be parented, and the support is not forthcoming.

The parents are also plagued by feelings of guilt vis-à-vis their own parents. One of the "tasks" of children is to produce grandchildren for their parents; it is part of an implicit and sometimes explicit compact that parents and children have. When the parents have a child with a disability, causing the grandparents pain instead of joy, the parents may feel guilty. Anger very often masks the guilt that the parents feel, and an unhealthy dynamic begins to develop in the parent–grandparent relationship.

Grandparents' feelings parallel closely the parents' responses. They feel grief, anger, anxiety, and guilt in varying proportions. They display their feelings to their children and to professionals in accordance with the cultural values of their family. More often than not, there is no openness about feelings between grandparents and parents. Frequently, neither wants to burden the other with their pain; they are very protective of each other. Unfortunately, this can be misinterpreted as indifference. Grandparents can be mistakenly viewed as being cold and uninvolved, when in reality they are frightened and concerned but very diffident about sharing their feelings. The parents and grandparents often need help in bridging the gap between them.

In the Emerson College program, we always try to provide a support group for grandparents, who are usually the most isolated and loneliest family members. It is often difficult to assemble enough grandparents to have a group, since many grandparents now live long distances from their children and grandchildren and visit only intermittently. Nevertheless, we make the attempt every year by scheduling a nursery day on a Saturday, long in advance and in the spring, when grandparents are more likely to return to the north, in the hope that we can gather enough grandparents for a group. I really enjoy a grandparent group, not only because I can relate so well to them since we are at similar life-cycle points, but also because of how lonely they are and how much they need support from us and from each other.

Occasionally all the grandparents live in our local area. When this happens, we offer the group an evening meeting in which I use the fishbowl design. Groups such as these almost invariably spark a great deal of family dialogue. They are also the most professionally satisfying groups that I lead.

The effects of the child with a disability on the parent–grandparent relationship do not have to be negative. Occasionally we have found the grandparents to be more capable than the parents, and they have assumed the primary caretaker role. They respond like parents, the only difference being that they are somewhat older and wiser; they are generally quite delightful to work with. They do wrestle with guilt that their child cannot assume the responsibility of raising the deaf child; they often see this as a failure on their part.

Parents frequently discover, after they have worked through their pain and anger, that the child's grandparents are an important resource for them, although not in the way that they had originally expected. Grandparents frequently provide respite care via very necessary babysitting so that parents can have some time out. Grandparents can also provide necessary parenting to the other siblings in the family when the parents are overwhelmed by the demands of the child with a disability. The surrogate parent role played by the grandparents can become very important for the emotional well-being of the nondisabled siblings. The restructured relationship between the parent and grandparent, once the parent gets through the existential crisis, can also be very exciting. For the first time, the parents can begin to feel and respond as adults with their own parents and, in turn, find themselves being treated as adults.

Siblings

Siblings are enormously important for the development of social skills. Within the sibling system, children learn how to resolve conflicts and how to be supportive of one another. They learn how to make friends and allies, how to save face while losing, and how to achieve recognition for their skills. The sibling system teaches children to negotiate, cooperate, and compete. The jockeying for position within the family system shapes and molds children into their adult models. When children come in contact with the world outside the family, they take with them the knowledge they learned from their siblings to form their peer relationships (Minuchin, 1974).

The sibling relationship is potentially the longest relationship in our lifetime. In some families this relationship is fostered and strong; in others it is very weak. Siblings also serve to validate each other's growing-up experiences. No two children are ever born into the same family, but the closest thing to someone who shares our cultural heritage is a sibling.

There is little in the literature about the effects of a child with a disability on the sibling system. Probably the most definitive study was by Grossman (1972), who tested and interviewed 83 college students who had siblings with developmental delay; she found that 90% of the subjects were affected by their siblings with developmental delays. The 10% of the subjects who were not affected were the oldest male children. The most affected were the oldest sisters, who were expected to participate in child-rearing activities and to assume many parental functions. In most families, there are different role expectations for oldest sons and oldest daughters. All younger siblings were affected one way or another by the child with a mental disability. The effects on the siblings were both negative and positive; in fact, the group of subjects split evenly, with 45% feeling that overall it was a negative experience and 45% feeling that it was a positive one.

The following negative consequences were noted by Grossman:

1. Shame about the sibling with developmental delay, and guilt about that shame.

2. Guilt about being in good health while the sibling is not.

3. A sense of being tainted or defective; concern that they themselves might have mental disability or might bear children with disability.

4. Guilt about having negative feelings toward the sibling who has a mental disability.

5. A feeling of having been neglected by the parents.

6. A feeling of having lost their own childhood because of the too-early assumption of responsibilities.

7. A belief that the sibling with a mental disability had put stress on the parental relationship, which negatively affected the rest of the family.

The positives for the siblings were the following:

1. Greater understanding of people in general and people with disabilities in particular.

2. More compassion.

3. More appreciation of their own good health and intelligence.

4. More sensitivity to prejudice.

5. A sense that the experience had drawn the family together.

6. A sense of vocational purpose and direction. (Many siblings become teachers of children with special needs.)

As one might expect, Grossman (1972) found that the more open and comfortable the parents were in talking about and accepting the child's disability, the better able the nondisabled sibling was to deal with it. When the parents accepted the child with a disability, they tended to help the nondis-abled child also come to a healthy acceptance. This finding has strong clinical implications for professionals working with children with disabilities because by working with the parents, as system theory would predict, they can also be working with the sibling system. The other finding that needs to be emphasized is that as tragic as having a disabled child may be, it can and does have a very positive effect on some families and the children within the families.

Seligman and Lobato (1983) reviewed earlier studies done on the non-disabled siblings of children with special needs. They concluded that there is a differential effect and called for longitudinal and better controlled studies. I fully concur with this finding.

There are few studies of siblings within the field of communication disor-ders. All the studies I have found are within the field of deafness; one wonders how siblings of children with speech and language disorders fare. My experi-ence would lead me to believe that there is no disorder-specific response and that all siblings will respond in pretty much the same way, depending on the cues they receive from their parents.

Schwirian (1976) interviewed 29 mothers of families in which there was a preschool child with a hearing impairment with older siblings, as well as 28 mothers of families with only nondisabled children. She found that older non-disabled siblings of children with hearing impairment had greater care respon-sibilities and fewer social activities than older siblings in the control group. Sisters had significantly higher child-care and overall responsibility scores than brothers, again indicating the different role expectations that parents have for sons and daughters. A major procedural weakness of the study is that she did not interview or test the siblings. Her data are only as good as the mothers are as observers of their children's feelings and behavior; in some cases, mothers' perceptions may not be very accurate. Mothers tend to not want to see the sib-ling pain, knowing that in many cases it was their inability to provide support that caused the pain.

Using self-report questionnaires, Israelite (1986) tested 14 hearing female adolescents (mean age of 16 years 3 months) who were the older sisters of chil-dren with hearing impairment and a matched group of 14 adolescents who had nondisabled siblings. She found that the two groups of older siblings differed significantly on only two traits: self-concept identity and social self. The results suggested that the hearing siblings defined themselves not only as individuals in their own right but as sisters of children with hearing impairment.

Darius (1988) interviewed siblings of children with hearing impairment. Her data indicated that siblings from small families, especially those with only two children, are most at risk for social and emotional difficulty. Siblings who are of the same gender and who are within 2 years of age of the deaf sibling are also at risk. Her data supported the notion that how well the parents accepted and adapted to the deafness was the major variable in the siblings' acceptance.

For my book *Deafness in the Family* (Luterman, 1987), I interviewed some of the original families that had gone through the Emerson College program. In one family, the oldest daughter had become a speech pathologist in Hawaii. I asked her to write about her experiences growing up with a deaf brother. I think her letter, printed below, poignantly illustrates the problems of the hearing sibling.

Dear Dr. Luterman:

I have been very busy this spring with work, my two special education classes that I am taking at the University of Hawaii, and the new group that I joined called Sign Express. It is a group of about 15 people that sign songs and put on performances to help educate others about sign language.

I am real excited about the book you are writing and I wish that I could have been there to talk with you when you went over to my family's house. I have a lot of feelings about Robert's deafness and how it has affected me. I have only told my mother some of my feelings because she gets upset or angry when I say how I felt when I was little. I don't know if it's because she thinks that I am saying that she was not a good mother to me, or why she gets upset.

I think when I was little, I had very mixed feelings. I felt very jealous of Robert but I also felt very proud of him. I can remember feeling very neglected, because I always thought that he got all of the attention from everybody. Of course now I realize that my mother had to work with him more and it was all necessary, but I didn't understand that when I was little. I remember wishing that I was deaf for a while, thinking that then I would get more attention. I remember wishing that I would get sick and have to go into the hospital so that everyone would bring me presents and give me more attention. I even remember trying to break my arm by jumping out of my treehouse (which never happened). I have never told my mother any of this. But I never hated Robert. I guess the way I dealt with my jealousy was by deciding to work with deaf children when I grew up. I decided this ever since I used to go watch Robert at Emerson College through the one-way mirror with my mother. And here I am, a speech pathologist working at a school where the deaf total communication class is housed, and I love working with the deaf kids (ages 5–12).

I also remember being very proud of Robert. I can remember going to his school plays at the school for the deaf and having tears come to my eyes when I watched him on stage. I remember wanting to be friends with his friends there. I also remember people saying mean things about deaf people in general, like they can't talk and they are all "deaf and dumb," and feeling so hurt and intimidated that I couldn't even stand up for deaf people. I usually just said nothing.

I guess Robert's deafness probably created a lot of extra tension in my parents' marriage. I remember my mother getting really upset about the taxis taking him to school, some school problem, and other things. I remember my father not wanting to or just not getting involved and my mother getting upset at him. I really never understood just how it affected my father but I know it was real hard on my mother. I never really noticed what effect Robert's deafness had on Lynda, Michael, or Nicole [siblings]. I didn't get along with Lynda, Michael, or Robert that much when I was little. Now I am much closer to everyone in my family.

Maybe it's because I live so far away I am trying to learn to sign fluently. Robert prefers to sign now and doesn't associate with hearing people if he can help it. Last summer when I went home for a visit, I played the card game Uno with Robert and his friends. At first I felt uncomfortable, but it was a lot of fun and I think that was the first time anyone in our family associated with him when he had his friends over. I wish I could spend more time with him and really get to know him. I have been able to get a hold of a TTY a few times and I love being able to talk to him over the phone. I always felt bad when I called home on holidays and could talk to everyone and then just be able to tell someone to say hi to Robert. I remember a couple of times he would get on the phone to say hi to me and then my mother would get on the phone and say "that was Robert," like I couldn't tell. I remember when we used to watch TV when we were little and Robert would always ask us what was going on in the show and we would get irritated at him and tell him to wait for the commercials. I wish we knew how to sign then and be able to interpret for him so he could understand while the show was on. I have very strong feelings about total communication. Robert has told me a lot about how he always felt left out and that makes me feel so sad for him because if we only used sign language he would have been more involved and would have known what was going on. But I realize that is a big issue that probably never will be solved.

Well I guess I rambled on quite a bit. I hope that this information will be helpful to you. If you have any more questions, please feel free to write to me. I'll be glad to help in any way possible. I would love to visit you the next time I get back to Boston and also visit the clinic at Emerson College.

Thank you for asking about my feelings.

How often do we ask siblings how they feel or include them in what we do? They can be immensely helpful in conducting diagnostics and in administering therapy. I often use them as test models for their siblings with hearing impairment. In the nursery program, we always set aside several days each semester specifically for siblings. On these days, the hearing children are allowed into the nursery and the therapy sessions. We give them a hearing test so that they know what takes place in a test suite. We are always very careful to ask them if there is something they want to know. Very often the siblings are our future speech pathologists and audiologists.

The solution to the sibling problem is easy to grasp intellectually and very hard to implement practically. Parents need to direct attention to the sibling as a person, not merely as a vehicle to produce a well-functioning child with a disability or as an impediment to that mission. Means must be found within the family for the sharing of feelings, and siblings must be given a chance to discuss their feelings of anger and guilt. Unfortunately, a fair balance is not easy to achieve, especially in the early years, as the parents do not have much energy and time for themselves, let alone for the nondisabled siblings. Parents frequently can identify the problem; however, because of limited resources, they cannot implement a solution. Here the grandparents can be very helpful. Also, paradoxically, if we can teach parents to take care of themselves, they will have energy and time left to share with the nondisabled siblings. Parents don't always see that it is not the quantity of time they spend as much as it is the quality.

Optimal Families

When we broaden our view from individual therapy to family therapy as proposed here, we in effect become a member of the family. As a member of the family, we teach by modeling effective behavior. For us to do this, we need to have a grasp of what it is we are working toward to help the family become more optimal. Several models of the optimal family have appeared in the family literature (Beavers & Voeller, 1983; Epstein, Bishop, & Baldwin, 1982; Olson, Russell, & Sprenkle, 1983; Trivette & Dunst, 1990). From these studies I have distilled the following five characteristics of the optimal family.

1. *Communication among all family members is clear and direct.* Almost any family therapist who has written about families has examined the communication patterns in the family. Invariably, dysfunctional families have dysfunctional communication pat-

terns. Using modeling, therapists encourage clear communication. Optimal families do not hold back or talk around an issue. Implicit expectations are always made explicit. Comments are always directed toward the person for whom they are intended. Talking is efficient and straightforward. Messages are congruent, containing both content and feelings. Empathy and humor characterize the communication among family members.

2. *Roles and responsibilities are clearly delineated, overlapping, and flexible.* An optimal family must have clear intergenerational boundaries, as well as a delineated sibling subsystem. The parents must have clear authority, and other roles in the family are allocated on the basis of ability rather than the basis of age or gender. Roles need to be overlapping as well, so that if one member of the family is not present, others can fill in. The children's responsibilities need to be altered as they grow, and responsibilities need to be renegotiated periodically. There must be a basis and structure for negotiation of role allocation. Optimal families allow for change in roles as needed to maintain a well-functioning unit.

3. *The family members accept limits for the resolution of conflict.* Conflict in families is normal and healthy; growth and change occur out of conflict. Parent–child and sibling relationships are inherently conflictual. In dysfunctional families, conflict is repressed; the family might appear harmonious, but when conflict does emerge, it becomes destructive. In optimal families, disputes are resolved in a way that is mutually satisfactory, and there is always a face-saving formula for any "loser." Conflict in an optimal family usually involves everyone winning. For example, the mother is about to cut a cake, and the two children are squabbling over who is going to get the bigger piece of cake. The mother lets one child cut the cake and lets the other child choose the first slice; the other child will cut the next cake, and the first child will choose the first slice. Children need to see that solutions are fair and that individual needs are always considered. Parents must also model conflict resolution for their children as the professionals model it for the parents.

4. *Intimacy is prevalent and is a function of frequent, equal-powered transactions.* One basic function of the family is to provide an environment where members feel loved. Families have different ways of expressing love. Some express this love physically through hugging and kissing, whereas others use more subtle expressions of caring. The caring needs to be communicated in such a way that the other family members can receive it. An optimal family provides intimacy while also respecting the need for space and distance. Optimal families are cohesive without being enmeshed.

5. *A healthy balance exists between change and the maintenance of stability.* The maintenance of stability is known as *homeostasis*. Families maintain their balance by making minute adjustments, much as a high-wire performer oscillates movements to stay on the wire (Harvey, 1989). Families must change to accommodate the life cycle. For example, the children age and make new demands on the parental restrictions; meanwhile, the parents age and are less adept at managing their lives, so other family members must fill

the void. Then there are the vicissitudes of life when a family is thrown a "curve ball." This happens when parents get ill, when an economic catastrophe occurs such as the loss of a job, or when a child is born with a disability. Optimal families are able to make the necessary changes while maintaining stability. Dysfunctional families are not able to accommodate to the change, and often dissolve or become so dysfunctional that they need massive amounts of external support.

The delicate balance between homeostasis and accommodating to change involves all of the other factors involved in an optimal family. Change can be accomplished best where there is open and clear communication among the family members, and where role flexibility enables others to step in to accommodate the increased demands of family time. There needs to be caring among the family members, and the family needs to have a means of dealing with the conflict that is inevitable any time there is a need for change.

Optimal families produce optimally functioning children and adults with disabilities. Our job as professionals in working with persons with communicative disorders is to help the family become optimal, or as close to it as possible. We can teach parents, mainly by modeling, how to manage conflict, how to communicate openly and honestly with their children, and how to display their affection and caring for their children. In effect, what we must do is parent the parents, which creates for them in our relationship an optimal clinical family. The parents then can take from our optimal clinical family the information and skills necessary for their own home situation.

The Successful Family

The notion of the optimal family is basically theoretical, stemming from the experience of family therapists working with dysfunctional families. There is some research on the successful family. The design of these studies was basically the same: The professionals working with the families rated the families as to their degree of success in coping with a child with a disability. Based on the ratings, the investigators then categorized families as successful, adequate, or inadequate. These families were then interviewed to determine the outstanding characteristics that led to the professional judgment. Gallagher et al. (1981) examined families in which there was a child with developmental delay; Lavell and Keogh (1980) examined families in which there was a child with diabetes; and Venters (1981) studied families in which there was a child with cystic fibrosis. The results of these studies suggest that the following four characteristics seem to underlie a successful family. These characteristics are very much in agreement with my own observations of the families of deaf children.

1. *A successful family is one that feels empowered.* Families need to feel that what they are doing will make a difference. Even with children having cystic fibrosis, a terminal illness, the parents need to feel that by working with the children they can prolong their lives and make their current living easier. I frequently see professionals who present such a bleak and hopeless picture to these parents that the parents never get over the feeling of "What's the use?" These families are never successful; we must never take away hope.

Parents are often rendered impotent by too much help from professionals. Sandow and Clarke (1977) studied the effects of a home intervention program on the performance of preschool children severely affected with Down syndrome and severe cerebral palsy. The 32 children in the study were divided into two matched groups. One group was visited by a therapist once every 2 weeks for a 2-hour session, whereas the other group was visited only once every 2 months. The study was conducted for 3 years, and at the end of each year the children were tested for their cognitive functioning and speech and language development. The findings were startling. Initially the more frequently visited children showed more gains in intellectual functioning and growth in speech and language than the less frequently visited children. By the second year of the study, the results reversed, with the less frequently visited children demonstrating more improvement than the more frequently visited children. By the third year, the gap had increased even further, demonstrating that less professional intervention was better than more. The researchers interpreted their data to suggest that parents in the less frequently visited group were less dependent on the therapist than were the more frequently visited parents. In short, they were empowered in that they were forced to rely on their own skills and strengths because they had a minimum of professional help.

My bias about home intervention programs is that they should be almost entirely parent centered and that the teachers should interact minimally with the child. The parent should do the lesson, and the teacher's role is one of coach or collaborator, and the teacher should focus on those things that the parent is doing well. The help provided by the teacher to the parent needs to be covert if the parent is to be empowered.

2. *In successful families the self-esteem, especially of the mother, is high.* This notion is very much related to the empowering notion discussed above. I think that the single most potent clinical intervention we can make to help a young client with a disability is to bolster the self-esteem of the parents, especially the mother. There is research justification for this notion. In a hallmark study, Schlessinger (1994) followed 40 families with a deaf child on a longitudinal basis for 20 years. She found that the best predictor of third-grade literacy was the self-esteem of the parents. This variable transcended hearing loss, methodology, and socioeconomic status. Similar results were reported by DesJardin et al. (2006) for families in which the child had a cochlear implant; parental efficacy was the key ingredient for success. This means that every clinical intervention that we perform needs to be evaluated in terms of whether it enhances the self-esteem

of the parents. Efficacy of our clinical interventions is going to be a matter of parental self-esteem.

When parents feel confident and empowered, they no longer need denial as a coping strategy. They are then able to work with the professional as coequals, and when this happens, the child benefits immensely. In the same vein, when working with adult clients, professional attention needs to be directed at empowering and increasing the self-confidence of the nondisabled spouse.

Therapists need to set up situations whereby the parents can experience some success in working with their children, especially in the early stages of the parent–professional interaction. As Featherstone (1980) so eloquently wrote, "Fears ease as experience discredits fantasy, as mothers and fathers learn that actual problems of raising their child differ from the ones they imagined. Similarly, small victories over private demons reassure parents about their own ability to raise their child" (p. 27).

3. *In successful families there is a feeling that the burden is shared.* In most families, one person, usually the mother or the nondisabled spouse, is designated as the primary caretaker for the person with a disability. If the rest of the family provides no support and respite care, the designated caregiver begins to feel resentful and martyred. When this happens, there is very little likelihood of a successful outcome. Other family members need not be overt in their help, but they need to be emotionally supportive of the caretaker and also willing to assume some of the other family responsibilities, freeing the caretaker to provide the direct therapy. This can occur even in a single-parent home if there is a feeling of a supportive network around the primary caretaker. Friends and other family members can fill in for the missing parent. Dundon, Carmer, and Novak (1987) found that the two major variables determining the success of families coping with Alzheimer's disease were health of the well spouse and the amount of unpaid help available to the family. When the well spouse felt supported by the community, the family coped successfully.

The family also needs to feel that the larger community is supportive and sharing the burden. In the initial diagnostic stages with a young child, the parents feel totally responsible. I often tell them, "This business is really in thirds—one third is your responsibility, one third is mine as a professional, and one third is the child's. You just be sure that you do your third, I'll do my third, and both of us will see that the child does his third."

4. *Successful families need to make philosophical sense of the situation.* All of us have a cosmology that is our way of explaining why and how things happen, especially why bad things happen. It is hard for most of us to accept the existential notion of randomness or the concept that we live in a world without meaning. So people seek an answer to the question, "Why me?" Not having a suitable answer may leave us stuck in bitterness and anger, which seldom leads to a successful outcome. Each family must come up with its own answer, which means that we as professionals sometimes need to get into uncomfortable areas of discussion as people come to grips with their own explanation

of why the terrible thing happened to them. For example, in one support group, a parent of a deaf child said, "Since this happened, I have stopped going to church," and a mother sitting opposite her said, "Since this happened, I've been going to church every day." A very fruitful discussion then ensued, as the parents worked through their feelings about "God" and reworked their religious views. In my clinical experience, the parents who show the least grief are the deeply religious ones. They see the disability as God's will, and although they cannot divine God's intention, they see themselves as his instrument and seem to get to work constructively with a minimum of grief.

A very successful mother of two deaf children and one child who was severely brain damaged as a result of a car accident had this to say:

> I always think of myself as a very average person. I have no particular talent, no particular anything. I'm a very average-type person and I've been given three very special kids. Sometimes I talk to God and I say, "Why did you give these kids to me? Why didn't you give them to someone who was different?" and so then I think, all right, I was given these kids and maybe this is my thing in life. Maybe all I'm going to do in life is to get these kids into adulthood, and maybe this is how my salvation will be measured.

With an explanation, we can go on and work; without one, we are forever pondering the why. For me, having a wife with multiple sclerosis was a challenge to make something good happen out of an awful disease. There is a marvelous Zen saying: "When the learner is ready, the teacher appears." For me and my wife, multiple sclerosis was our teacher.

The stress on families, which is a reflection of both sociological changes and the change engendered by a person with a disability, is not necessarily a negative force. I have seen a great deal of growth occur as a result of this stress. Many siblings decide to become therapists. Although some marriages founder, others are strengthened. For the parents, the child with a disability can offer an opportunity to restructure a relationship that has gone stale. Men have often reported how delighted they were to find out how much strength their wives have; the wives were delighted with the caring qualities that emerged in their husbands. Often both parents have found a new purpose in working very hard together in parent organizations and therapy programs, thereby strengthening the bond between them.

Similarly, the parent–grandparent relationship can be restructured. For the first time, many parents begin to respond as adults to their own parents and, in time, find themselves being treated as adults. They often begin to see their own parents as vulnerable fellow adults, and that is very exciting.

For me there has always been growth in stress. I am pushed by the stress to develop more capacity in order to reduce the stress. I generally give to life what life demands. When life demands more, I am forced to expand. That increased capacity is my growth. I see this happening in all the families I have worked with. Although I can empathize and perhaps sympathize with the pain involved, I know that if they can just hang in, they will learn and grow. They have a powerful teacher in the disorder, and we as professionals must allow the process of growth to take place. We can facilitate the growth by not overhelping and by at all times respecting the dignity and the capacity of our clients to grow. Very often we have to let go of our preconceived notions. The following anonymously written poem has helped me with the necessary letting go.

To Let Go

To Let Go is not to stop caring,
It's recognizing I can't do it for someone else.
To Let Go is not to cut myself off,
It's realizing I can't control another.

To Let Go is not to enable,
But to allow learning from natural consequences.
To Let Go is not to fight Powerlessness,
But to accept the outcome is not in my hands.

To Let Go is not to try to change or blame others,
It's to make the most of myself.
To Let Go is not to care for, it's to care about.
To Let Go is not to fix, it's to be supportive.

To Let Go is not to judge,
It's to allow another to be a human being.
To Let Go is not to try to arrange outcomes,
But to allow others to affect their own destinies.

To Let Go is not to be protective,
It's to permit another to face their own reality.
To Let Go is not to regulate anyone,
But to strive to become what I dream I can be.

To Let Go is not to fear less, it's to love more.

COUNSELING AND THE FIELD OF COMMUNICATION DISORDERS

Educating the Clinician

During the 1960s, a notable attempt was made to define the field of speech–language pathology and audiology by giving it a narrow, technical base. This ensured our survival as an independent profession with a solid core of research expertise and scientific credibility. Now that we are established, we have been moving into a more humanistic, family-oriented field that borrows heavily from psychology, social work, and family therapy.

It presently appears that our training programs are lagging behind the needs of the field. As stated in Chapter 1, McCarthy, Culpepper, and Lucks (1986) surveyed the training programs accredited by the American Speech-Language-Hearing Association (ASHA). They found that only 40% of training programs offered a course in counseling within their department, 36% offered a course outside the department (over half of these courses were offered within psychology and education departments and had no content related to speech and hearing), and 23% offered no course in counseling. Only one third of the programs required students to take a counseling course, despite the fact that 70% of the respondents felt that counseling was a very important skill that should be offered within the program. The authors concluded their study with the following observation:

> Although the fields of audiology and speech–language pathology recognize counseling as an essential component of diagnostic and therapeutic procedures and as a professional responsibility, the emphasis training programs place on it may not reflect its importance. Students are often trained in counseling theory and techniques only when they have chosen to take such a course.

Even then, counseling specific to communication disorders is frequently not included. These data are underscored by the finding that only 12% of the respondents in this study felt that training programs are sufficiently preparing students to meet the counseling needs of individuals with communicative disorders. (p. 52)

The follow-up to that study has indicated no essential change in our field (Culpepper, Mendel, & McCarthy, 1994). To date, there is no further follow-up to the Culpepper et al. study; my sense is that there has not been much movement in the field. I, too, feel that we are not training our students appropriately to prepare them to meet the emotional demands of a helping profession. From the humanistic point of view, a client's learning and growth take place best in a nonthreatening atmosphere of warmth and acceptance. To facilitate this growth, the therapist needs to be a caring, nonjudgmental, congruent person. None of these skills is exotic; they are all within the purview of everyone. The job of the training program is to help develop these attributes in student clinicians. Unfortunately, almost all graduate training programs tend to stress students' intellectual and cognitive skills but not their interpersonal abilities. For example, selection of students is generally based on their intellectual skills as exemplified by Graduate Record Examination scores or grade-point averages. Rarely are interpersonal skills considered, except perhaps indirectly as reflected in letters of recommendation. However, the present era of full disclosure and threat of litigation has rendered letters of recommendation almost meaningless. The grade-point average seems to lend an objective measure that graduate schools can defend. Interpersonal skills are not readily measurable and may be difficult to defend if challenged by an irate student. The danger for our field in ignoring interpersonal skills, however, is very great; we can turn out students who are knowledgeable about the field but who are clinically and interpersonally inept.

It appears that graduate schools are selecting reasonably "normal" students. Crane and Cooper (1983) gave the *Minnesota Multiphasic Personality Inventory* (MMPI) to 130 female speech–language graduate students. The resultant profiles indicated that the students "were manifestly normal but rather passive, compliant, stereotypically feminine, sensitive, anxious" (p. 139). It concerns me that we are willing to accept these attributes as normal for women. I prefer to think that much of what we are viewing as "stereotypically feminine" is in reality a reflection of our teaching and attitudes toward women. I hope that this attitude is changing. I am deeply concerned about the passivity and compliance aspects of the personality profile, and what that bodes for our profession. In all fairness, Crane and Cooper also found that the students were highly imaginative, creative, and energetic and I have certainly met and worked with my share of students with these delightful characteristics. From the research of Miller and Potter (1982), however, we also know that many of these students will burn out at an alarming rate.

Training Students for Clinical Competence and Personal Growth

I am not sure that the MMPI measures some important personality variables that influence clinical competency. For example, the "Annie Sullivan" type of student needs to be identified early in his or her career. This type is a caring person with energy and a marvelous impulse to be helpful that can be directed, but we must provide experiences on the training level to increase self-awareness of the need to be needed. The Annie Sullivan types must learn how to help in a way that is truly helpful so that the client's self-esteem and independence are not compromised. Our personal satisfactions as professionals can come from knowing internally what we have done and not from receiving the approval of others. In short, we also have to help develop in students an inner locus of evaluation.

Occasionally we get interpersonally inept students who are otherwise very intelligent, and there needs to be a place within our profession for them. I think they can be helped to become more adept with some structured interpersonal experiences; they may also make good researchers.

Another kind of student occasionally gets through our screening process: the student with a limited capacity to care for others. I think that I can teach almost anything except the capacity to care. This student probably will be a professional disaster despite any technical skills we might teach, and we need to have better mechanisms to screen such students out of the profession.

If one examines closely the training of speech–language pathologists and audiologists, it is apparent that the training moves along poorly conceived behavioral lines. Control is generally external to the students: The teacher decides what the students need to know and rewards them if they appear to learn the material. Student clinicians also learn to please the supervisor, which also encourages the development of an external locus of evaluation. (No wonder they are passive and compliant!)

The communication disorders literature, on the other hand, does reveal a humanistic thread in the supervisory relationship. Ward and Webster (1965) urged that we treat our students as human beings, and that their self-actualization be an important consideration in the training program. They argued for courses within the curriculum that are geared to explain human behaviors and that can then be applied to students. Van Riper (1965) described the sometimes painful role of the supervisor:

> He is a friendly person looking on interestedly in what is taking place, warmly empathizing with the success and making no issue about the failures. Even when the student is demonstrating outrageous sins of omission or commission the supervisor does not seize the reins. He suffers silently and keeps a poker face and formulates what he will say to the clinician later. (p. 77)

Van Riper believed that we should treat the student clinician with the same loving respect that we wish him or her to accord the client.

Pickering (1977) argued that the student needs to have relationship skills as much as knowledge about the field. She stated that the supervisory relationship can be the vehicle for the student to learn about relationships and for promoting personal growth and change in both the supervisor and student clinician. The supervisory relationship needs to have the elements of authenticity, dialogue, risk taking, and conflict in order to facilitate student growth.

Caracciolo, Rigrodsky, and Morrison (1978) wrote that a supervisor should model the Rogerian, nondirective role to the students. The Rogerian relationship would have a high degree of unconditional regard, empathy, and congruence. The students, after experiencing the growth in this humanistic relationship with the supervisor, would in turn be able to foster this kind of relationship with their clients.

I agree with the premise of Caracciolo et al. (1978) that experiencing the humanistic relationship is the best way of learning it. The authors make me uncomfortable, however, when they state that "it is necessary to define operationally and construct specific training procedures that will develop among supervisors the necessary attitudes and skills that will contribute to personal and professional growth" (p. 290). It seems to me that when we set about "operationally defining" and "developing specific training procedures," we lose the essence of the humanistic approach. At some fundamental level, humanism is ineffable. True learning is an inside-out process; we must lead students to it and hope they find it by creating for them the right conditions of a growth-promoting relationship. When we deliberately structure the learning situation so as to teach techniques, we are imposing a cognitive solution on an affect problem. Students tend to learn the form of the humanistic approach but not the substance. (Anyone who has tried to have a conversation with a student who thinks that Rogerian reflective listening means repeating back the last thing the person has said begins to get an insight into the causes of homicide.)

Klevans, Volz, and Friedman (1981) attempted to train students in interpersonal skills. One experimental group was taught skills via extended role playing, having to assume the role of a person with a speech, language, or hearing impairment in an out-of-class assignment. The second group was required to observe clinical interactions and to code behavior. The authors found that the students in the experiential group were able to make significantly more facilitative verbal responses than the coding-observing group when tested in a simulated helping relationship. The authors felt that the total length of time (8¾ hours) devoted to training both groups was insufficient for mastering interpersonal skills.

I think this study points up several things that need to be examined. If we are going to train students in interpersonal skills, the experience needs to be hands-on rather than didactic. We cannot lecture within a class or even have students observe interactions and then expect them to be interpersonally adept. It is also clear that we have to allot more time within the curriculum for working on interpersonal skills. The 8¾ hours of time allotted in this study, which was part of a one-credit clinic practice course, is unfortunately typical of most training programs and rather pathetic for attempting to teach such fundamental clinical skills.

I think we also need to attack the problem from the personal growth side. We cannot limit our endeavors to teaching interpersonal skills from a strictly technical point of view. For me, the best way of teaching and learning counseling has been within the context of my own personal growth experiences, which have included such diverse activities as workshop attendance, immersion in sensitivity groups, and an Outward Bound learning experience where I had to rock-climb and sail. The latter experience was especially helpful; an underlying theme of that experience was, "We have met the enemy and found it is us." I have had to learn to give myself permission to think, to feel, and to be productive. Recently I have found that periodically going on a Buddhist retreat where much time is given to self-reflection is a valuable time-out for me. I have found that as I have come to accept myself more, I also accept and value others more.

The dilemma of the supervisory or teaching relationship in developing humanistic relationships with students is the evaluative function held by the teacher. As long as the supervisor or teacher has the power of the grade, locus of control is always external to the student, and authenticity on the student's part in relation to the supervisor is very hard to accomplish. At some level and at some time, the student must please the teacher in order to get a passing grade. It would require a very high degree of trust to develop authenticity in the relationship. True equality is not really possible because the levels of personal power are inherently unequal. Van Riper (1965) argued that we should be collaborators with our students rather than supervisors. This ideal is very hard to accomplish when the supervisors must give the students grades or eventually write letters of recommendation. Although the supervisors may feel that they are collaborators, the students feel differently, as one might expect. Culatta, Colucci, and Wiggins (1975) found wide discrepancies between the supervisor's and the student clinician's views of their relationship. In my supervisory work I encourage students at the inception of the semester to do it badly so then we can help them. By the end of the semester I expect them to be doing it well and I assure them that their grade will be a function of how well they do at the end of the semester. I also tell them something is only a mistake when they do it a second time. Somehow we must create the conditions of safety so that students are willing to risk and to reveal their inadequacies. This is especially hard to do at the graduate level, when students have learned so well how to "fake it."

In my teaching of content-level courses, I have attempted to work out a compromise between cognitive and interpersonal learning needs. At the beginning of the course, I give the students the final examination, which consists of a list of essay questions that reflect my opinion as to what content they need to master and from which I will select a number of questions for the actual final. I also give the students a bibliography containing readings that will enable them to find the answers to the questions. It is then the students' responsibility to organize their time to master that content. The grade for the course is based solely on the examination performance, and students are encouraged to be as ignorant as possible during class sessions. I comment that they should be ignorant; that's why they are taking the course. The only time they cannot afford to be "ignorant" is on the final examination. The Instructor's Manual on the disk that accompanies this text provides details on how I teach this course.

I usually take responsibility for structuring half of the class sessions with lectures, films, videos, or guest speakers. The students are required to structure the other half of the sessions. The unstructured sessions usually start out with painful silences until the students realize that nothing happens until they make it happen. Periodically we evaluate the class, and everyone, including myself, has a chance to talk about how things are going. Within this format, the students get a chance to obtain some control of what they learn; they have to take responsibility for obtaining content and are never required to read anything. Generally the course evaluations by the students are enthusiastic, although as we near examination time, their anxiety begins to increase and they begin to have regrets about their freedom. Because the students are not usually familiar with a learning situation in which they have to assume so much responsibility, they frequently use their time to meet the demands of other courses and find themselves far behind in our course. Bargaining sessions frequently ensue in which they try to limit the scope of the examination, delay the final, plead to make it a take-home exam, and so on. I delight in the give-and-take of the negotiations in which we engage, as it reflects equality and authenticity in our relationship. I generally remain tough; if the students are to learn responsibility assumption, they must not be let off the responsibility hook lightly.

My sense of teaching this way is that the students get as much, and often more, content than they did when I took sole responsibility for content. I also am astonished at the interesting byways of content that emerge out of the students' interests. For example, one of my aural rehabilitation classes decided to read Mark Medoff's (1981) play *Children of a Lesser God,* which involves the relationship between a deaf woman and a hearing male speech therapist. From the in-class play reading and discussion, the students obtained a great deal of insight into the problems of deaf–hearing relationships and of contemporary issues among deaf adults. The understanding obtained was of a much deeper dimension than they would have obtained from a review of the didactic literature alone.

Evidence in the literature suggests that locus of control can be shifted to a more internal orientation as a result of learning or teaching experiences. Johnson and Croft (1975) found that students enrolled in a personalized system of instruction (PSI) course demonstrated a statistically significant internally oriented shift as measured by the Rotter Locus of Control scale after the students completed the course. The PSI course has no midterm or final examination; it is entirely self-paced and self-graded. Performance is often evaluated in a personal interview. This sort of course can be modified to become a marvelous blend of behaviorist and humanist notions. Similarly based courses, which would include more contact with the teacher within a humanistic relationship, could be developed within the field of communication disorders in order to develop self-managing students who also have experienced a clinically and personally useful relationship with a teacher.

In these professionally perilous times of high burnout rate and declining student enrollment, we must find creative solutions to implementing humanistic-based education that encourages an inner locus of control. This is not to say that we should give up our cognitive and evaluative functions; we must supplement content with interpersonal learning. It is unreasonable to expect students trained within the current poorly conceived behavioral model to easily take responsibility for themselves and for the profession. The behavioral model, with its emphasis on external locus of control and external locus of evaluation, tends to produce professionals who will accept poor working conditions, work mechanically, and not take responsibility for furthering the profession—by passively and compliantly accepting things as they are. If we do not anticipate change and act, we will be overwhelmed by it. The future of our profession, I think, rests in altering our current educational practices to include a more humanistic base, which will in turn create a more self-confident, self-reliant, and assertive professional, one who will also be much more effective in serving persons with communication disorders. We owe our clients and our profession nothing less.

If there is going to be any meaningful change in the current parent–professional relationship, it will have to occur at the professional training level. Too many young clinicians leave their training programs with minimal or very inadequate experience in relating to clients' parents. I suspect that part of the problem lies in the lack of emphasis in parent training by the supervisors and academic teachers in their training programs. The current ASHA regulations (2003) allow 25 clock hours of student activity with parents to be counted toward the 375 hours needed for certification. There are no mandated family work or counseling requirements.

On a national level, we also need to promote continuing education workshops specifically geared toward professionals in academic programs on the utilization of parents in working with their children and the training of students in parent involvement. We need to increase the number and quality of parent involvement programs throughout the nation. Cartwright and Ruscello (1979) reported that only half of all approved clinics had a parent involvement program. Although this study is clearly dated, there is no evidence that the inclusion of parent programs has increased. This 50% figure seems inadequate to me, especially since nearly 90% of all programs report that parent involvement is very important (Cartwright & Ruscello, 1979). We should also be very concerned about the quality of the parent programming. There are too many professional-centered parent programs—that is, programs in which the professional has the control and uses the educational program to promote a particular point of view and in which the personal growth of the parents is minimal. A good parent program has to be designed with the parent in mind. If we try to append a parent program onto an existing child-centered program, we are doomed to failure. The program rapidly becomes the PTA model of parent involvement, which usually entails hurried parent conferences and lectures in which parents are *talked at* rather than *listened to*. In good programming, the parent is the primary target.

Good parent programs have a snowball effect. They produce self-confident, positively assertive parents who will work as equals with other professionals. These parents, in effect, become trainers of all professionals. They open the eyes of professionals to the potential of parent involvement. The reasonably self-confident professional finds it a relief to have a parent as a coworker.

If parent–professional relationships are to improve, they have to be freed from a problem-centered orientation. Much of the parent–professional contact occurs only when there is a specific problem. It is very hard to have a productive relationship when it is always problem centered. I give my aural rehabilitation class a role-playing situation in which a teacher of deaf students calls a parent to school to tell the parent that his or her child is "an oral failure" and should be put in a total communication program. The problem is set up to be adversarial in that the parent is strongly committed to an oral education. The situation usually ends up in disaster, in part because if this is the first parent–professional meeting (as generally happens), it is already too late. Time has not been spent in developing the necessary trust, autonomy, and initiative before the parent and professional can deal with such a loaded topic as changing the mode of communication for the child.

Some of my students solve this problem well. They recognize that the person with the problem is the teacher, not the parent or the child. When the teacher can convey to the parent that the teacher has a problem and can enlist the parent's help, then the relationship does not become adversarial. It is also agreed by the class after the role-playing activity that the teacher should have seen the parents outside of the school and established and worked on their relationship before any problems occurred.

Parents and professionals in speech–language pathology are natural allies. They both want in the most ardent terms the same thing: a child with better communicating skills. Murphy (1981), in an almost lyrically written and lovely book on parents, *Special Children, Special Parents*, wrote, "Parents and workers are sculptors helping to shape what a child may become. There is a place for all—a place to be, to become something more than they now are, a place to learn, to dance, to sing" (p. ix).

Professional Burnout

The problem of professional burnout in the helping professions is quite severe. Meadow (1981) administered a burnout inventory to 240 teachers of the deaf. Among the findings of her study were the following:

◆ Teachers of the deaf had a higher burnout rate than classroom teachers who were teaching children with normal hearing.

◆ Burnout was highest among teachers who had been working 7 to 10 years in the job and was lowest among teachers who had been working 11 or more years and among new teachers.

◆ Burnout was directly related to perceived ability to influence the work situation. Teachers who felt they had the power to influence their jobs showed the least burnout.

◆ Teachers who showed the highest personal involvement in their jobs also tended to have the highest burnout rate.

These results are very interesting. Greater stress appears to occur among professionals working with students with disabilities than among professionals working with students without disabilities. Young teachers seem to be carried through their first years by idealism and enthusiasm. From the Meadow (1981) data and from my own observation, many young beginning teachers get overinvolved with the students. Mattingly (1977) noticed this phenomenon among child-care workers: Burnout was signaled by workers who began to merge themselves and their lives with the institution. When this merging occurs, the individual loses the resources to give to others. A helping professional is very much like a gasoline station where people come to fill up. At some point, a truck comes and fills the tanks of the gasoline station. The professional who merges with the population he or she is serving is always among needy people and has little opportunity to "fill his or her own tank." I think that this is the one who burns out within that 7- to 10-year period.

Those professionals who survive beyond the 10-year period learn better coping strategies, probably because they have learned to meet their personal needs outside of their work experiences. Based on Meadow's (1981) data, it would also seem that they have a more internal locus of control than do the burnout sufferers, since burnout is directly related to the perceived inability to influence the work situation. Teachers with an inner locus of control are not "pushed into" accepting poor working conditions and are also more likely to assert themselves with administrators.

Within the context and terminologies of this book, burnout can be viewed as primarily a problem in dealing with the existential issue of loneliness and love: The need to be loved can push the teacher into an unwholesome, over-involved relationship with the students. Using the Erikson model, burnout can also be seen as an intimacy issue in that there is a fusion of the personal life and the job. I think that, overall, burnout is a locus-of-control problem because people who feel that they have no power, who are like "leaves in the wind," simply meeting other people's demands, will lose all feeling for their clients, will become emotionally exhausted and drained, and will burn out. To paraphrase the Dali Lama, "We all seek happiness but seldom practice its causes." When we take control of our happiness and practice its causes, we don't burn out; instead, we flourish.

I think that we can effect changes in the burnout phenomenon by providing ongoing workshops and inservice training for working professionals. I think that a more efficient way of dealing with this problem is for universities to focus on producing students who value themselves, who have an awareness of their own needs, who have an ability to be authentic in relationships, and who have a more internal locus of control and locus of evaluation. Also, it is a good idea for all professionals to guard themselves with flexibility and nourish themselves with humor to help prevent burnout.

Counseling Within the Public Schools

The public school setting is a difficult milieu for counseling to occur in. The typical therapy model for the public school setting is one in which the children are taken out of class for individual therapy. Because of caseload numbers, therapists sometimes offer therapy in small groups. Contact with the parents is usually minimal, sometimes just a phone call and more often simply messages carried back and forth by the child. It has always struck me that the underlying assumptions of this therapy model are incredibly naive. It assumes in effect that by working in isolation with the child for an hour a week (in some cases for only half an hour), a therapist can significantly alter the child's communication skills. It presupposes an incredibly powerful effect of individual therapy. It also burdens the child to be the change agent for the whole family system.

I think many therapists in the public schools intuitively recognize the absurdity of their professional lives, wherein they have huge caseloads and inadequate help and facilities. The restrictions they have accepted, either because those restrictions have been externally imposed or because of an internal reluctance to risk changing them, do not allow the therapists to do an effective job. When that happens, they either leave their positions quickly or they burn out and go through the motions of the job knowing full well that they are being ineffective.

I think there are ways to restructure jobs so that therapists become effective change agents. Therapists need to see themselves as consultants/counselors rather than as direct purveyors of therapy. Therapy, where possible, needs to be directed at the caregivers in order to be more effective. Within the public school setting, the teachers have the parental role. We as therapists can be much more efficient if we alter the classroom environment, which is the child's home away from home, so that it becomes more facilitative for the development of good communication skills for all the children. This means we must spend our time with the teachers in the classroom, or with the parents helping them to help the children with communication disorders.

I think this consultative model of speech pathology is slowly taking hold and will become the dominant therapeutic model. Superior and Leichook (1986) strongly recommended a parent consultant model within the public school setting. They suggested that

> parent meetings could be scheduled in lieu of the child's treatment sessions providing that the goal of parent consultation be addressed within the individual education plan. A few parent meetings may, in fact, have far greater effect than several therapy sessions. (p. 402)

My sense is that the time spent with parents or teachers is usually the most fruitful time, and the thrust of therapy needs to be at the teacher or parent level. My preference is to use the term *collaborative* as opposed to *consultive*; collaborative implies an equality of relationship and is empowering, in contrast to consultive, which implies the professional as the expert.

In setting up the collaborative model, it is critical that the therapist, before initiating any direct therapy with the child, meet with the classroom teachers and the child's parents. At this time a clear contract needs to be drawn up that specifies the expectations of everyone. I think the therapist needs to move toward a contract with the parents and the teachers that requires them to have some direct involvement in the therapeutic process. The contract has to be flexible, and opportunities must be provided for renegotiation. If there is any failure to meet contractual expectations, then the teacher or parent has to be called on the carpet. It is absolutely essential that a working relationship be established before the initiation of therapy. This establishes the basis for any ongoing disputes involving the child directly or the contractual obligations.

One of the primary opportunities for parents and therapists to interact is during the development of the child's Individualized Education Program (IEP). In poorly run school programs, the process is usually painful for the parents, as they are subjected to professionals' reports in an arena-style conference. Parents usually leave intimidated and more confused than they were going into the conference, and certainly not empowered. Andrews and Andrews (1993) presented a model of developing an educational plan that serves to empower parents, and I think this model needs to be adopted widely. In their approach, which is family centered, all members of the family are encouraged to participate. The families are listened to and encouraged to participate actively in the assessment of the child. The authors presented enabling techniques adapted from family therapy approaches that are readily within the grasp of professionals who work with persons with communication disorders.

Multiculturalism

Van Kleeck (1994) described the many cultural traps that the insensitive speech–language pathologist can fall into. For example, when the speech–language pathologist assumes that getting the child to initiate more communication means getting the child to initiate conversation with adults, he or she may be unwittingly violating a family norm. In many cultures, children are not encouraged to initiate conversations with adults. The danger is ever present that we might impose our cultural values on others. It is so easy to operate from our own ethnocentric perspective that we fail to appreciate cultural differences.

On the other hand, there is an equal danger that in looking for cultural differences among populations, we might fall into the trap of cultural stereotyping. Within any cultural grouping, there are always variations in behavior, and the generalizations we might make about a population may not apply to the specific individual with whom we are working. What needs to be understood is that in one sense we are all multicultural; each family must be approached as a marvelous experiment of one. We must take each family and each individual within the family as they come and allow them to teach us the best way for them to learn. We always need to respect the dignity of each family we encounter, and as Van Kleeck (1994) pointed out, we must create an educational program to fit the family rather than try to fit the family to our program. This notion undergirds everything that is in this text. By listening to and valuing our clients, we will always respect their unique cultural heritage, and clients and families will tell us the best way for them to be taught.

The Limits of Counseling

In a thoughtful article, Stone and Olswang (1989) tried to define the boundaries for counseling by speech–language pathologists and audiologists. They argued that many times the problem is not that we need better counseling skills, but that the client should be referred to a mental health professional. The boundary for this referral is very hard to define, and Stone and Olswang failed to offer clear guidelines. I am not sure I have any clear guidelines either. I have found that as I have become more comfortable with myself and more comfortable with affect in my relationships, my professional boundaries have expanded and

I am willing to allow my professional relationships much greater latitude. I no longer refer clients. Instead I tell them that where we are is outside my scope of practice and leave it there. Generally clients then refer themselves. It is very difficult to refer a client to a mental health professional in such a way that does not provoke extreme anxiety in the client. The message being sent to the client, no matter how nicely worded, is that the problem is so formidable that he or she needs to see someone else. This is often very threatening to clients because the idea of emotional problems in many families carries a severe stigma.

I believe that in many cases the speech–language pathologist or audiologist should not be tempted to make a referral to mental health professionals, but instead should work to improve his or her own skills. I think psychologists and social workers who are employed in clinics need to provide ongoing inservice training to speech–language pathologists and audiologists to help them increase their counseling skills and confidence in their ability to relate on the affect level with clients. This requires the mental health professional to be professionally secure and able to accept a consultative role. Unfortunately, there are many "Annie Sullivan" psychologists and social workers who are anxious to rescue the speech–language pathologist or audiologist; this "de-skills" them in the same way that Annie de-skilled Mrs. Keller.

Undoubtedly, there are people with emotional disturbance who develop communication disorders or who are the relatives of someone with a communication disorder. These people are not normally upset, although they may seem so at the beginning, but are truly emotionally disturbed and have a multitude of life adjustment problems. I think speech–language pathologists and audiologists have a responsibility to identify these clients and then to set firm boundaries.

Counseling skills permeate everything I do. I do not want us or expect us as a profession to charge for "counseling." This is something a mental health professional does, and it would be an inappropriate professional invasion for us to do so. What we need to be doing is infusing counseling notions in everything we do. Many of the problems we encounter with clients can be solved by using techniques culled from the family therapy literature. Stone (1992) demonstrated how a systems approach can be used to analyze problematic relationships so as to improve the interactions between the professional and the families involved in the therapy. As mentioned previously, Andrews and Andrews (1993) used systems theory to help empower families during the IEP process. I think this trend will continue as we discover and utilize material and techniques garnered from the psychotherapy literature.

I think the key to counseling is the congruence of the counselor. As I become more congruent, technique slips away or, more accurately, becomes incorporated into everything I do. I think the most important thing a counselor brings to the helping relationship is self. The importance of the congruent professional far exceeds the value of any diagnostic test or specific techniques in counseling. If the literature on the desirable personality characteristics of the counselor were examined, it would appear that no one would qualify unless one could also qualify for sainthood. May (1989) noted that one outstanding characteristic of the successful counselor is the "courage of imperfection," meaning the ability to fail. He also indicated that the successful counselor is one who is interested in people for their own sake. It is not necessary to be an entirely self-actualized person to be an effective counselor; rather, I think one needs to have a deep interest in people and sensitivity to others. One needs to be a caring individual who does not impose beliefs on others, who maintains a constant awareness of self, and who does not hide behind the artificiality of being a professional. Before encountering a client, Carl Rogers used to pray, "Please let me be sufficient." And so sufficient is enough. Our growth as a profession will be measured by how we grow as individuals. We owe our profession and our clients our commitment to learn about ourselves as well as our field; we can do no less.

REFERENCES

Albertini, J., Smith, J., & Metz, D. (1983). Small group versus individual speech therapy with hearing impaired young adults. *Volta Review, 85*, 83–87.

Alpiner, J. (1978). Ancillary personnel in rehabilitation. In S. Alpiner (Ed.), *Handbook of adult rehabilitative audiology* (pp. 232–274). Baltimore: Williams & Wilkins.

American Speech-Language-Hearing Association. (2003). *Knowledge and skills acquisition (KASA) summary form for audiology.* Retrieved August 24, 2007, from http://www.asha.org

American Speech-Language-Hearing Association. (2006). *Roles, knowledge, and skills: Audiologists providing clinical services to infants and young children birth to 5 years of age.* Retrieved July 30, 2007, from http://www.asha.org/docs/html/KS2006-00259.html

Andrews, M. A. (1986). Application of family therapy techniques to the treatment of language disorders. *Seminars in Speech and Language, 7*, 347–358.

Andrews, M., & Andrews, J. (1993). Family-centered techniques: Integrating enablement into the IFSP process. *Journal of Childhood Communication Disorders, 15*(1), 41–46.

Arbuckle, D. S. (1970). *Counseling: Philosophy, theory and practice* (2nd ed.). Boston: Allyn & Bacon.

Asha Interview: Geri Jewell. (1983). *Asha, 25*, 18–22.

Backus, O., & Beasley, J. (1951). *Speech therapy with children.* Cambridge, MA: Houghton Mifflin.

Bardach, J. (1969). Group sessions with wives of aphasic patients. *International Journal of Group Psychotherapy, 119*, 361–366.

Baumgarten, M., Battista, R., Infante-Rivard, M., Hanley, J., Becker, R., & Gauthier, S. (1990). The psychological and physical health of family members caring for an elderly person with dementia. *Journal of Clinical Epidemiology, 45*(1), 61–70.

Beavers, R., & Voeller, M. (1983). Comparing and contrasting the Olson Circumplex Model with the Beavers Systems Model. *Family Process, 22*, 85–98.

Berry, J. O. (1987). Strategies for involving parents in programs for young children using augmentative and alternative communication. *Augmentative and Alternative Communication, 3*(2), 90–93.

Bodner, B., & Johns, J. (1977). Personality and hearing impairment: A study in locus of control. *Volta Review, 79*, 362–368.

Bynner, W. (Trans.). (1962). *The way of life according to Lao-tze.* New York: Capricorn Books.

Byrne, M. (2000). Parent-professional collaboration to promote spoken language in a child with severe to profound hearing loss. *Communication Disorders Quarterly, 21*(4), 210–223.

Caracciolo, G., Rigrodsky, S., & Morrison, E. (1978). A Rogerian orientation to the speech-language pathology supervisory relationship. *Asha, 20*, 286–290.

Cartwright, L., & Ruscello, D. (1979). A survey on parent involvement in speech clinics. *Asha*, *21*, 275–280.

Cassell, E. J. (1999). *The nature of suffering and the goals of medicine*. New York: Oxford University Press.

Cole, S., O'Conner, S., & Bennett, L. (1979). Self-help groups for clinic patients with chronic illness. *Primary Care*, *6*(2), 325–339.

Coles, R. (1970). *Erik H. Erikson: The growth of his work*. Boston: Little, Brown.

Cook, J. (1964). Silences in psychotherapy. *Journal of Counseling Psychology*, *11*, 42–46.

Cooper, E. (1966). Client-clinician relationships and concomitant factors in stuttering therapy. *Journal of Speech and Hearing Disorders*, *9*, 194–199.

Cottrel, A., Montague, J., Farb, J., & Throne, S. (1980). An operant procedure for improving vocabulary definition performance in developmentally delayed children. *Journal of Speech and Hearing Disorders*, *45*, 90–95.

Craig, A., Franklin, J., & Andrews, G. (1985). The prediction and prevention of relapse in stuttering. *Behavior Modification*, *9*, 422–442.

Crane, S., & Cooper, E. (1983). Speech-language clinician personality variables and clinical effectiveness. *Journal of Speech and Hearing Disorders*, *48*, 140–147.

Crowley, M., Keane, K., & Needham, C. (1982). Fathers: The forgotten parents. *American Annals of the Deaf*, *127*, 38–45.

Culatta, R., Colucci, S., & Wiggins, E. (1975). Clinical supervisors and trainees: Two views of a process. *Asha*, *171*, 152–156.

Culpepper, B., Mendel, L., & McCarthy, P. (1994). Counseling experience and training offered by ESB-accredited programs. *Asha*, *36*, 55–64.

Dale, P. (1991). The validity of a parent report measure of vocabulary and syntax at 24 months. *Journal of Speech and Hearing Research*, *34*, 565–571.

Darius, B. (1988). A study of siblings of hearing impaired children: How they were affected by the handicap. Unpublished master's thesis, Emerson College, Boston.

Davies, H., Priddy, M., & Tinkleberg, J. (1986). Support groups for male caregivers of Alzheimer's patients. *Clinical Gerontologist*, *5*, 385–394.

Dee, A. (1981). Meeting the needs of the parents of deaf infants. *Language, Speech and Hearing Services in Schools*, *12*, 13–21.

DesJardin, A., Eisenberg, L., & Hodapp, R. (2006). Supporting families of young deaf children with cochlear implants. *Infants and Young Children*, *19*(3), 179–189.

Dowaliby, E., Burke, N., & McKee, B. (1983). A comparison of hearing impaired and normally hearing students on locus of control, people orientation, and study habits and attitudes. *American Annals of the Deaf*, *128*, 53–59.

Dundon, M., Carmer, S., & Novak, C. (1987). *Distress and coping among caregivers of victims of Alzheimer's disease*. Paper presented at the annual meeting of the American Psychological Association, New York.

Edgerly, R. (1975). The effectiveness of parent counseling in the treatment of children with learning disabilities. Unpublished doctoral dissertation, Boston University.

Egolf, D., Shames, G., Johnson, P., & Kasprisin-Burrell, S. (1972). The use of parent interaction patterns in therapy for young stutterers. *Journal of Speech and Hearing Disorders*, *37*, 222–227.

Ellis, A. (1977). The basic clinical theory of rational-emotive therapy. In A. Ellis & R. Grieger (Eds.), *Handbook of rational-emotive therapy* (pp. 11–19). New York: Springer.

Emerick, L. (1988). Counseling adults who stutter: A cognitive approach. *Seminars in Speech and Language, 9*, 257–267.

Emerson, R. (1980). Changes in depression and self-esteem of spouses of stroke patients with aphasia as a result of group counseling. Unpublished doctoral dissertation, Oregon University, Eugene.

Epstein, N., Bishop, D., & Baldwin, L. (1982). McMaster model of family functioning: A view of the normal family. In E. Walsh (Ed.), *Normal family process* (pp. 148–172). New York: Guilford Press.

Erikson, E. H. (1950). *Childhood and society* (2nd ed.). New York: Norton.

Farran, C., Keane-Hagerty, E., Salloway, S., Kupferer, S., & Wilken, C. (1991). Finding meaning: An alternative paradigm for Alzheimer's disease family caregivers. *The Gerontologist, 31*, 483–489.

Featherstone, H. (1980). *A difference in the family.* New York: Basic Books.

Flahive, M., & Schmitt, M. (2004, February). Counseling and the school based speech-language pathologist. *Advance*, pp. 10–12.

Flahive, M., & White, S. (1982). Audiologists and counseling. *Journal of the Academy of Rehabilitative Audiology, 10*, 275–287.

Fleming, M. (1972). A total approach to communication therapy. *Journal of the Academy of Rehabilitative Audiology, 5*, 28–35.

Friehe, A., Bloedow, A., & Hesse, S. (2003). Counseling families of children with communication disorders. *Communication Disorders Quarterly, 24*(4), 211–220.

Fromm, E. (1941). *Escape from freedom.* New York: Holt, Rinehart & Winston.

Gallagher, J. J., Cross, A., & Scharfman, W. (1981). Parental adaptation to a young handicapped child: The father's role. *Journal of the Division for Early Childhood, 3*, 3–14.

Gath, A. (1977). The impact of the abnormal child upon the parents. *British Society of Psychiatry, 130*, 405–410.

Ginsberg, A., & Wexler, K. (1999). Understanding stuttering and counseling clients who stutter. *Journal of Mental Health Counseling, 22*, 228–239.

Girolametta, M. E., Greenberg, J., & Manolson, A. (1986). Developing dialogue skills: The Hanen Early Language Parent Program. *Seminars in Speech and Language, 7*, 367–382.

Gregory, H. (1983). *The clinician's attitudes in counseling stutterers* (Publication No. 18). Memphis, TN: Speech Foundation of America.

Grossman, E. K. (1972). *Brothers and sisters of retarded children.* Syracuse, NY: Syracuse University Press.

Haas, W. H., & Crowley, D. S. (1982). Professional information dissemination to parents of preschool hearing-impaired children. *Volta Review, 84*, 17–23.

Haggard, R., & Primus, M. (1999). Parental perceptions of hearing loss classification in children. *American Journal of Audiology, 8*, 1–10.

Hallahan, P., Gasar, A., Cohen, S., & Tarver, S. (1978). Selective attention and locus of control in learning disabled and normal children. *Journal of the Learning Disabled, 11*, 47–57.

Hanh, T. N. (1999). *The heart of the Buddha's teaching.* New York: Broadway Books.

Hansen, J., Stavis, R., & Warner, R. (1977). *Counseling theory and process*. Boston: Allyn & Bacon.

Harris, S., Handiman, J., & Palmer, C. (1985). Parents and grandparents view the autistic child. *Journal of Autism and Developmental Disorders, 15*, 125–135.

Harvey, M. (1989). *Psychotherapy with deaf and hard of hearing persons: A systemic model*. Hillsdale, NJ: Erlbaum.

Hinkle, S. (1991). Support group counseling for the caregivers of Alzheimer's disease patients. *The Journal for Specialists in Group Work, 16*, 185–190.

Hoffman, L. (1981). *Foundations of family therapy*. New York: Basic Books.

Holland, A. (2006). Living successfully with aphasia: Three variations on the theme. *Top Stroke Rehabilitation, 13*(1), 44–51.

Holt, J. (1964). *How children fail*. New York: Dell.

Hornyak, A. (1980). The rescue game and the speech-language pathologist. *Asha, 22*, 86–94.

Israelite, N. K. (1986). Hearing impaired children and the psychological functioning of their normal hearing siblings. *Volta Review, 88*, 47–54.

Johnson, W., & Croft, R. (1975). Locus of control and participation in a personalized system of instruction course. *Journal of Educational Psychology, 67*, 416–421.

Kabat-Zinn, J. (2005). *Wherever you go, there you are: Mindfulness meditation in everyday life*. New York: Hyperion Books.

Kazak, A., & Marvin, R. (1984). Differences, difficulties and adaptations: Stress and social networks in families with a handicapped child. *Family Relationships, 33*, 67–77.

Klevans, D., Volz, H., & Friedman, R. (1981). A comparison of experimental and observational approaches for enhancing the interpersonal communication skills of speech-language pathology students. *Journal of Speech and Hearing Disorders, 46*, 208–212.

Kommers, M. S., & Sullivan, M. D. (1979). Wives' evaluation of problems related to laryngectomy. *Journal of Communicative Disorders, 12*, 411–418.

Kopp, S. (1972). *If you meet the Buddha on the road, kill him!* Palo Alto, CA: Science and Behavioral Books.

Kopp, S. (1978). *An end to innocence*. New York: Bantam.

Kornhaber, C., & Woodward, L. (1985). *Grandparents/grandchildren The vital connection*. New Brunswick, NJ: Transaction Books.

Kubler-Ross, E. (1969). *On death and dying*. New York: Macmillan.

Land, S. L., & Vineberg, S. E. (1965). Locus of control in blind children. *Exceptional Child, 31*, 257–263.

Lash, J. V. (1980). *Helen and teacher*. New York: Delacorte.

Lavell, N., & Keogh, B. (1980). Expectation and attribution of parents of handicapped children. In S. S. Gallagher (Ed.), *Parents and families of handicapped children* (pp. 48–72). San Francisco: Jossey-Bass.

Lear, M. (1980). *Heartsounds*. New York: Simon & Schuster.

Lerner, W. (1988). *Parents' and audiologists' perspectives regarding counseling*. Unpublished master's thesis, Emerson College, Boston.

Lieberman, M., Yalom, I., & Miles, M. (1973). *Encounter groups: First facts*. New York: Basic Books.

Lloyd, L., Spradlin, J., & Reid, M. (1968). An operant audiometric procedure for difficult-to-test patients. *Journal of Speech and Hearing Disorders, 33*, 236–242.

Lobato, D. (1983). Siblings of handicapped children: A review. *Journal of Autism and Developmental Disabilities, 13*, 347–364.

Lowe, T. (1989). *Grandparents view the hearing impaired child.* Unpublished master's thesis, Emerson College, Boston.

Lund, N. J. (1986). Family events and relationships: Implications for language assessment and intervention. *Seminars in Speech and Language, 7*, 415–436.

Luterman, D. (1969). Hypothetical families. *Volta Review, 71*, 347–351.

Luterman, D. (1979). *Counseling parents of hearing-impaired children.* Boston: Little, Brown.

Luterman, D. (1987). *Deafness in the family.* Boston: Little, Brown.

Luterman, D., & Kurtzer-White, E. (1999). Identifying hearing loss: Parents' needs. *Journal of Audiology, 8*, 8–13.

Madison, L., Budd, K., & Itzkowitz, J. (1986). Changes in stuttering in relation to children's locus of control. *Journal of Genetic Psychology, 147*, 233–240.

Malone, R. L. (1969). Expressed attitudes of families of aphasics. *Journal of Speech and Hearing Disorders, 34*, 146–151.

Martin, E., Krueger, S., & Bernstein, M. (1990). Diagnostic information transfer to hearing-impaired adults. *Texas Journal of Audiology and Speech Pathology, 16*(2), 29–32.

Maslow, A. H. (1962). *Towards a psychology of being.* Trenton, NJ: Van Nordstrand.

Massie, R., & Massie, S. (1973). *Journey.* New York: Knopf.

Matis, E. (1961). Psychotherapeutic tools for parents. *Journal of Speech and Hearing Disorders, 26*, 164–170.

Matkin, N. (1998). The challenge of providing family-centered services. In T. Bess (Ed.), *Children with hearing impairment: Contemporary trends.* Nashville, TN: Vanderbilt University Press.

Matson, D., & Brooks, L. (1977). Adjusting to multiple sclerosis: An explorative study. *Social Science and Medicine, 11*, 245–250.

Mattingly, M. A. (1977). Sources of stress and burnout in professional child care work. *Child Care Quarterly, 6*, 127–130.

Maxwell, D. (1982). Cognitive and behavioral self-control strategies: Applications for the clinical management of adult stutterers. *Journal of Fluency Disorders, 7*, 403–432.

May, R. (1989). *The art of counseling.* Lake Worth, FL: Gardner Press.

McCarthy, P., Culpepper, N., & Lucks, L. (1986). Variability in counseling experiences and training among ESB accredited programs. *Asha, 28*, 49–53.

McKelvey, J., & Borgersen, M. (1990). Family development and the use of diabetes groups: Experience with a model approach. *Patient Education and Counseling, 16*, 61–67.

Meadow, K. (1981). Burnout in professionals working with deaf children. *American Annals of the Deaf, 126*, 13–19.

Medoff, M. (1981). *Children of a lesser god.* New York: James T. White.

Mendelsohn, M., & Rozek, E. (1983). Denying disability: The case of deafness. *Family Systems Medicine, 1*(2), 37–47.

Miller, M., & Potter, R. (1982). Professional burnout among speech-language pathologists. *Asha, 24*, 177–180.

Minuchin, S. (1974). *Families and family therapy.* Cambridge, MA: Harvard University Press.

Minuchin, S., Rosman, B., & Baker, L. (1978). *Psychosomatic families.* Cambridge, MA: Harvard University Press.

Mitford, J. (1963). *The American way of death.* New York: Simon & Schuster.

Moore, P. (1982). Voice disorders. In G. Shames & E. Wiig (Eds.), *Human communication disorders* (pp. 312–346). Columbus, OH: Merrill.

Moustakes, C. (1961). *Loneliness.* Englewood Cliffs, NJ: Prentice Hall.

Munro, J., & Bach, T. (1975). Effect of time limited counseling on client change. *Journal of Counseling Psychology, 22*, 395–406.

Murphy, A. (1981). *Special children, special parents.* Englewood Cliffs, NJ: Prentice Hall.

Murphy, A. (1982). The clinical process and the speech-language pathologist. In G. Shames & E. Wiig (Eds.), *Human communication disorders* (pp. 386–402). Columbus, OH: Merrill.

Nuland, S. D. (1994). *How we die.* New York: Knopf.

Olson, D., Russell, C., & Sprenkle, D. (1983). Circumflex model of marital and family systems: VI. Theoretical update. *Family Process, 22*, 69–83.

Pearlin, L., & Schooler, S. (1978). The structure of coping. *Journal of Health and Social Behavior, 19*, 2–21.

Peck, S. (1978). *The road less traveled.* New York: Simon & Schuster.

Pedersen, F. (1976). Does research on children reared in father absent families yield information on father influences? *Family Coordinator, 25*, 459–463.

Perkins, W. P. (1977). *Speech pathology: An applied behavioral science* (2nd ed.). St. Louis: Mosby.

Pickering, M. (1977). An examination of concepts operative in the supervisory process and relationship. *Asha, 19*, 697–770.

Post, J. (1983). I'd rather tell a story than be one. *Asha, 25*, 22–25.

Rabins, P. (1984). Management of dementia in the family context. *Psychosomatics, 25*, 369–375.

Rimm, D. C., & Cunningham, H. M. (1985). Behavior therapies. In S. J. Lynn & J. P. Garske (Eds.), *Contemporary psychotherapies* (pp. 44–70). Columbus, OH: Merrill.

Robertson, E., & Suinn, R. (1968). The determination of rate of progress of stroke patients through empathy measures of patient and family. *Journal of Psychosomatic Research, 12*, 189–193.

Rogers, C. (1951). *Client-centered therapy.* Boston: Houghton Mifflin.

Rogers, C. (1980). *A way of being.* Boston: Houghton Mifflin.

Rollins, W. (1988). Counseling spouses of the communicatively impaired. *Seminars in Speech and Language, 9*, 269–277.

Rotter, S. (1966). Generalized expectancies for internal versus external control of reinforcement. *Psychology Monographs: General and Applied, 1*(Whole No. 609).

Roy, R. (1990). Consequences of parental illness on children: A review. *Social Work and Social Sciences Review, 2*(2), 109–121.

Sabbeth, B., & Leventhal, J. (1988). Trial balloons: When families of ill children express needs in veiled ways. *Children's Health Care, 171*, 87–92.

Sager, C. (1978). *Marriage contract and couple therapy*. New York: Rawson, Wade.

Sandow, S., & Clarke, D. B. (1977). Home intervention with parents of severely subnormal, preschool children: An interim report. *Child Care, Health and Development, 4*, 29–39.

Satir, V. (1967). *Conjoint family therapy*. Palo Alto, CA: Science & Behavior Books.

Schein, J. (1982). Group techniques applied to deaf and hearing-impaired persons. In M. Seligman (Ed.), *Group psychotherapy and counseling with special populations* (pp. 41–60). Baltimore: University Park Press.

Schlessinger, H. (1994). The elusive X factor: Parental contributions to literacy. In M. Walworth, D. Moones, & T. O'Rourke (Eds.), *A free hand* (pp. 37–66). Silver Spring, MD: TS Publishers.

Schlessinger, H., & Meadow, K. (1971). *Deafness and mental health: A developmental approach* (Rep. No. RD283-S). Washington, DC: U.S. Department of Health, Education, and Welfare.

Schwirian, P. (1976). Effects of the presence of a hearing impaired preschool child in the family on behavior patterns of older "normal" siblings. *American Annals of the Deaf, 121*, 373–380.

Seligman, M. (1982). *Group psychotherapy and counseling with special populations*. Baltimore: University Park Press.

Seligman, M., & Lobato, D. (1983). Siblings of handicapped persons. In M. Seligman (Ed.), *The family with a handicapped child: Understanding and treatment* (pp. 3–27). New York: Grune & Stratton.

Shames, G., & Florance, C. (1982). Disorders of fluency. In G. Shames & E. Wag (Eds.), *Human communication disorders* (pp. 86–110). Columbus, OH: Merrill.

Shirlberg, L., Diabless, D., Carlson, K., Filley, F., Kwiatkowski, J., & Smith, M. (1977). Personality characteristics, academic performance and clinical competence in communication disorders majors. *Asha, 19*, 311–315.

Shlien, J., Mosak, H., & Dreikors, R. (1962). Effects of time limits: A comparison of the psychotherapies. *Journal of Counseling Psychology, 9*, 31–36.

Singler, J. (1982). The stroke group: Planning for success. In M. Seligman (Ed.), *Group psychotherapy and counseling with special populations* (pp. 170–196). Baltimore: University Park Press.

SKI-HI Communicative Disorders Institute [National Summer Conference]. (1985). Ogden: Utah State University.

Skinner, B. F. (1953). *Science and human behavior*. New York: Macmillan.

Starkweather, C. (1974). Behavior modification in training speech clinicians: Procedures and implications. *Asha, 16*, 607–612.

Stech, E., Curtiss, J., Troesch, P., & Binnie, C. (1973). Clients' reinforcement of speech clinicians: A factor analytic study. *Asha, 15*, 287–291.

Stone, J. (1992). Resolving relationship problems in communication disorders treatment: A systems approach. *Language, Speech and Hearing Services in Schools, 23*, 300–307.

Stone, J., & Olswang, L. B. (1989). The hidden challenge in counseling. *Asha, 31*, 27–30.

Superior, K., & Leichook, A. (1986). Family participation in school based programs. *Seminars in Speech and Language, 7*, 395–414.

Sweetow, R. (1999). *Counseling for hearing aid fitting*. San Diego: Singular Press.

Tanner, D. C. (1980). Loss and grief implications for the speech-language pathologist and audiologist. *Asha, 22*, 916–922.

Tattersall, H., & Young, A. (2006). Deaf children identified through newborn hearing screening: Parents' experiences of the diagnostic process. *Child Care, Health and Development, 32*(1), 33–45.

Trivette, C., & Dunst, C. (1990). Assessing family strengths and family functioning style. *Topics in Early Childhood Special Education, 10*(1), 16–20.

Vance, B. (1998). Stroke! This isn't the script I was writing! In W. Sife (Ed.), *Enhancing the life* (pp. 149–160). New York: Haworth Press.

Van Kleeck, A. (1994). Potential cultural bias in training parents as conversational partners with their children who have delays in language development. *Asha, 35*, 67–76.

Van Riper, C. (1965). Supervision of clinical practice. *Asha, 7*, 75–78.

Venters, M. (1981). Familial coping with chronic and severe childhood illness: The case of cystic fibrosis. *Social Science and Medicine, 15A*, 289–297.

Ventimiglia, R. (1986). Helping couples with neurological disabilities: A job description for clinical sociologists. *Clinical Sociology Review, 4*, 123–139.

Ward, B., & Webster, E. (1965). The training of clinical personnel: A concept of clinical preparation. *Asha, 7*, 103–108.

Webster, E. (1966). Parent counseling by speech pathologists and audiologists. *Journal of Speech and Hearing Disorders, 31*, 331–345.

Webster, E. (1968). Procedures for group counseling in speech pathology and audiology. *Journal of Speech and Hearing Disorders, 33*, 27–35.

Webster, E. (1977). *Counseling with parents of handicapped children*. New York: Grune & Stratton.

Webster, M. (1982). *Hear Here Newsletter of the Canadian Speech and Hearing, 6*, 235–237.

White, K. (1982). Defining and prioritizing the personal and social competence needed by hearing impaired students. *Volta Review, 84*, 266–273.

Williams, D. M. L., & Derbyshire, J. O. (1982). Diagnosis of deafness: A study of family responses and needs. *Volta Review, 84*, 24–30.

Wright, D. (1969). *Deafness*. New York: Stein & Day.

Yalom, I. (1975). *The theory and practice of group psychotherapy*. New York: Basic Books.

Yalom, I. (1980). *Existential psychotherapy*. New York: Basic Books.

Yalom, I. (1989). *Love's executioner*. New York: Basic Books.

Yarnell, G. (1983). Comparisons of operant and conventional audiometric procedures with multi-handicapped (deaf-blind) children. *Volta Review, 85*, 69–74.

Zeine, L., & Larson, M. (1999). Pre- and post-operative counseling for laryngectomees and their spouses: An update. *Journal of Communication Disorders, 32*, 51–71.

INDEX

Acceptance, 71–72
Ackerman, Nathan, 146
Adolescence, 162–163
Affect response in counseling, 97–98
Affirmation
  as coping stage, 71
  as counseling technique, 100
Albertini, J., 124
Allen, Woody, 19
Alpiner, J., 150
Altruism, 14, 126
Alzheimer's disease, 124, 164–166
American Cancer Society, 123
American Speech-Language-Hearing Association (ASHA), xvii, 2, 8–9, 181–182, 188
Andrews, G., 109
Andrews, J., 192, 194
Andrews, M., 149, 192, 194
Anger
  in client–professional relationship, 60–61
  as healthy emotion, 61
  of parents or spouses, 58–61, 157–158
  of professionals, 65–66
  in teacher–parent relationship, 61
Aphasia, 149–150
Arbuckle, D. S., 15, 94
ASHA. See American Speech-Language-Hearing Association (ASHA)
Audiologists. See also Counseling
  certification of, 188
  counseling skills of, 2–3
  diagnosis by, 77–91
  emotions of, 65–68
  group process used by, 123–124
  and limits of counseling, 193–195
  parent programs and, 188–189
  training and education for, 2, 181–189
Augmentative and alternative communication systems, 148
Autistic children, 95

Autonomy
  communication disorders and, 38
  in counseling, 41–42
  versus shame and doubt (Erikson model), 34–35

Bach, T., 24
Backus, O., 17, 124
Baker, L., 147
Baldwin, L., 174
Bardach, J., 124, 149
Baumgarten, M., 165
Beasley, J., 17, 124
Beavers, R., 174
Behavior modification, 13–14
Behavioral counseling
  application of, to communication disorders, 13–14
  compared with other counseling approaches, 31–32
  description of, 11–13, 94
  limitations of, 14–15
Bennett, L., 124
Bernstein, M., 2, 78
Berry, J. O., 148
Binnie, C., 14
Bishop, D., 174
Bloedow, A., 53
Bodner, B., 108
Borgersen, M., 124
The Bourgeois Gentleman (Moliere), 23
Bowen, Murray, 146
Brain damage, 25, 179
Brooks, L., 67
Budd, K., 109
Buddhism, xviii, xix
Burke, N., 108
Burnout, 189–191
Bynner, W., 15
Byrne, M., 148

Cancer patients, 19–20
Caracciolo, G., 17, 184
Carmer, S., 178
Cartwright, L., 188
Case studies, 102–107
Cassell, E. J., xviii
Catharsis, 127–128
Changing-topic silence, 112–113
Cheerleading, 121–122
Childhood and Society (Erikson), 33
Children of a Lesser God (Medoff), 187
Chodren, Pema, xix
Clarke, D. B., 177
Cleft palate, 25, 89
Client-centered collaborative diagnosis, 79–91
Client-Centered Therapy (Rogers), 15–16
Cognitive therapy
    applications of, to communication disorders,
        29–30
    compared with other counseling approaches,
        31–32
    description of, 28–29, 94
    limitations of, 30–31
    rational-emotive therapy, 28–29
Cohen, S., 109
Cohesiveness of groups, 127
Cole, S., 124
Coles, Robert, 33
Colucci, S., 186
Communication disorders. See also Counsel-
        ing; Diagnosis; Emotions; and specific
        disorders
    anger and, 58–61
    behavioral counseling and, 13–14
    causes of, 87
    cognitive therapy and, 29–30
    confusion and, 63–65
    emotions of, 51–75
Erikson's life cycle model and, 38–39
    existentialism and, 23–27
    grief and, 52–55, 83, 84
    groups in speech–language pathology and
        audiology, 123–124
    guilt and, 62
    humanistic counseling and, 16–17
    inadequacy feelings and, 55–58
    locus of control and, 108–111
    vulnerability and, 62–63
Conflict

in families, 175
in groups, 138–139
Confrontation, 133–134, 137–138
Confusion, 63–65
Congenital diagnosis, 89–91
Congruence
    of client, 6–7
    of counselors, 16
Content response, 95–96
Contracting, 113–114
Control. See Locus of control
Cook, J., 112
Cooper, E., 17, 182–183
Coping process
    affirmation stage, 71
    denial stage, 67–70, 80, 82, 86
    flight strategy for, 72–73
    integration stage, 71–72
    modification strategy for, 73
    reframing strategy for, 74
    resistance stage, 70–71
    stress reduction and, 74–75
Cottrel, A., 13–14
Counseling. See also Counseling techniques;
        Emotions; Group process
    autonomy and, 41–42
    behavioral counseling, 11–15, 94
    cognitive therapy, 28–31, 94
    definition of, 7
    diagnostic process and, 77–91
    effectiveness of, 115–116
    emotions of communication disorders and,
        8–9, 51–75
    existentialism and, 18–27, 94
    family counseling, 145–150
    generativity and, 48
    humanistic counseling, 15–18, 94
    identity and, 45–47
    industry and, 43–45
    by informing, 1–4, 64–65
    initiative and, 42–43
    integrity and, 48–49
    intimacy in, 47
    limits of, 193–195
    by listening and valuing, 6–9
    medical model of, 1–6
    mistakes in, 51–52, 86, 115, 118–122
    multiculturalism and, 193
    by persuading, 4–6, 31

in public school settings, xvi, 3–4, 191–192
skills of audiologists and speech-language
    pathologists in, 2–4
termination phase of, 48, 139–140
theories of, 11–32
training and education in, 2, 181–189
trust and, 40–41, 97
Counseling techniques
affect response, 97–98
affirmation, 100
case studies, 102–107
changing-topic silence, 113
cheerleading as pitfall, 121–122
content response, 95–96
contracting, 113–114
counselor control via response, 94–102
counselor feedback, 114–115
counterquestion, 96–97
deciding how to respond, 100–102
denial misunderstood as pitfall, 121
effectiveness of, 115–116
implicit expectations as pitfall, 120
introduction to, 93–94
locus of control, 108–110
mistakes in, 51–52, 86, 115, 118–122
over–helping as pitfall, 24–25, 57–58, 121,
    183, 194
professional humility, 116–117
projection as pitfall, 119–120
reflective silence, 113
reframing, 98–99
sharing self, 99–100
silence, 111–113
stereotyping as pitfall, 119
termination silence, 113
transference as pitfall, 119
unattractive clients, 118
Counterquestion, 96–97
Craig, A., 109
Crane, S., 182–183
Credibility of therapists, 40–41
Croft, R., 187
Cross, A., 155
Crowley, D. S., 3
Crowley, M., 161
Culatta, R., 186
Culpepper, B., 2, 182
Culpepper, N., 2, 181–182
Cunningham, H. M., 12
Curtiss, J., 14

Dale, P., 81
Dali Lama, 118, 190
Darius, B., 171–172
Davies, H., 124
Deaf children. See also Communication disorders
behavioral therapy for, 14
congenital diagnosis of, 89–91
Erikson's life cycle model and, 38–39
locus of control and, 108
low expectations of, 24
mother's appreciation of father of, 162
parents of, 2–3, 4, 179
Deafness in the Family (Luterman), 172–173
Death, 19–20, 23–24
Death fantasies, 73
Dee, A., 4, 56, 124
Deferred diagnosis, 79–89
Dementia, 124, 164–166
Demonstration (teaching device), 43, 44–45
Denial
as coping strategy, 67–70, 80, 82, 86
misunderstanding of, by counselor, 121
as response to diagnosis, 80, 82, 86
Derbyshire, J. O., 2, 79
DesJardin, A., 149, 177
Despair versus ego integrity, 37
Diagnosis
and cause of disorder, 87
client-centered collaborative diagnosis, 79–91
by committee, 78
congenital or sudden inception diagnosis, 89–91
deferred diagnosis, 79–89
denial and, 80, 82, 86
information provided following, 83, 86–87
institution-centered diagnosis, 77–79, 89-91
interpersonal, affective dimension of, 82–89
medical model of, 77–78
parents' involvement in, 80–88
steps in, 88–89
Divorce, 72–73, 159
Doubt versus autonomy, 34–35, 38, 41–42
Dowaliby, E., 108
Down syndrome, 89, 157
Dreikors, R., 24
Dundon, M., 178
Dunst, C., 174
Edgerly, R., 148
Education. See Training in counseling
Education of the Handicapped Act Amend-
    ments of 1986 (P.L. 99-457), 150

Ego integrity
  counseling and, 48–49
  versus despair (Erikson model), 37
Egolf, D., 147–148
Eisenberg, L., 149
Ellis, Albert, 28–29, 110
Emerick, L., 29
Emerson, R., 124, 149
Emerson, Ralph Waldo, 21, 118
Emerson College, xvii, 78, 138, 157, 159–162, 168
Emotions
  affect response by counselor, 97–98
  allowing and eliciting feelings in counseling, 7–9, 52
  anger, 58–61, 157–158
  of clients, 51–65
  confusion, 63–65
  coping process and, 67–75
  diagnosis and, 82–89
  of grandparents, 168
  grief, 52–55, 83, 84, 158–159
  group process and affect release, 129
  guilt, 62, 158, 168
  inadequacy, 55–58
  mistakes in counseling involving, 51–52, 86, 115
  of parents, 8–9, 157–159
  of professionals, 65–67
  of siblings, 170, 172–174
  vulnerability, 62–63
Empathic listening, 16, 97
Empowerment of families, 177
Epstein, N., 174
Erikson, E. H.
  biographical information on, 33
  life cycle model of, 33–49, 190
  writings by, 33
Escape from Freedom (Fromm), 21
Existentialism
  application of, to communication disorders, 23–27
  compared with other counseling approaches, 31–32
  counseling and, 18–27
  death as issue of, 19–20, 23–24
Erikson's life cycle model and, 49
  freedom/responsibility as issue of, 20–21, 24–25
  group process and, 128
  issues of, 19–23, 94
  limitations of, 27
  loneliness as issue of, 21–22, 25–26
  meaninglessness as issue of, 22–23, 26–27
  vulnerability and, 62–63
Families. See also Parents
  case studies on, 102–107
  characteristics of successful families, 176–180
  components of, 151–174
  conflict in, 175
  counseling with, 145–150
  diagnosis and, 80–88
  divorce and, 72–73, 159
  empowerment of, 177
  grandparents in, 166–169, 179
  intimacy in, 175
  optimal families, 174–180
  and philosophical sense of disability, 178–179
  sharing of burden within, 178
  siblings in, 169–174
  spouses in, 58–61, 151–154
  stress in, 179–180
Family counseling, 145–150. See also Families
Farb, J., 13–14
Farran, C., 23
Featherstone, H., 157, 178
Feedback by counselor, 114–115
Feelings. See Emotions
Fialka, Janice, 84–86
Flahive, M., xvi, 1, 3–4
Fleming, M., 150
Flight strategy for coping, 72–73
Florance, C., 13
Fluency disorders. See Stutterers
Frankl, Viktor, 18
Franklin, J., 109
Freedom/responsibility, 20–21, 24–25
Freud, Anna, 33
Freud, Sigmund, 12, 33
Friedman, R., 184–185
Friehe, A., 53
Fromm, Erich, 18, 21

Gallagher, J.J., 155, 176
Gasar, A., 109
Gath, A., 157
Generativity
  counseling and, 48
  versus stagnation (Erikson model), 37
Ginsberg, A., 124
Girolametta, M. E., 149

Grandparents, 166–169, 179
Gravina, Gian Vincenzo, 113
Greenberg, J., 149
Gregory, H., 7
Grief
    episodic notion of, 53–54
    of parents, 48, 52–55, 83, 84, 158–159
Grossman, E. K., 169–171
Group process
    affect release and, 129
    altruism and, 126
    catharsis and, 127–128
    cohesiveness and, 127
    conflict and, 138–139
    confrontation and, 133–134, 137–138
    content and, 128–129, 139
    curative factors in, 125–128
    existential issues and, 128
    and filling available time, 142–143
    goals of, 128–129
    here-and-now norm and, 134
    homogeneity of grouping, 141–142
    hope and, 125
    inception stage of group, 136–138
    information provided through, 125–126
    initiative norm and, 132
    interaction norm and, 131–132
    interpersonal learning and, 126–127
    introduction to, 123
    leadership in, 130–135
    personal growth and, 129
    procedural norms and, 135
    resistance and, 138
    respect for individual needs and, 134–135
    self-disclosure and, 132–133
    size and setting of group, 142
    in speech–language pathology and audiology,
        123–124
    stages of group development, 135–140
    structured experiences and, 140–141
    termination stage of group, 139–140
    universality and, 125
    working group stage, 138–139
Guilt
    and institutionalization of parent with demen-
        tia, 165
    of parents, 62, 158, 168
    of professionals, 66
    of siblings, 170
    versus initiative (Erikson model), 35, 42–43

Haas, W. H., 3
Haggard, R., 2
Hallahan, P., 109
Handiman, J., 167
Hanh, T. N., xviii
Hansen, J., 32
Harris, S., 167
Harvey, M., 175
Hearing aid evaluation, 145–146
The Heart of the Buddha's Teaching (Hanh), xviii
Here-and-now norm, 134
Hesse, S., 53
Hinkle, S., 124
Hodapp, R., 149
Hoffman, L., 146, 147
Holland, A., 21
Holt, J., 45
Homeostasis, 175–176
Homogeneity of grouping, 141–142
Hope, 125
Hornyak, A., 24
Humanistic counseling
    application of, to communication disorders,
        16–17
    compared with other counseling approaches,
        31–32
    description of, 15–16, 94
    limitations of, 17–18
    professional humility, 116–117
    training in, 184
Humility of professional, 116–117

Identity
    communication disorders and, 38–39
    counseling and, 45–47
    versus role confusion (Erikson model), 35–36
IEP (Individualized Education Program), 78, 192
If You Meet the Buddha on the Road, Kill Him!
        (Kopp), 15
Implicit expectations, 120
Inadequacy, feelings of, 55–58
Inception stage of group, 136–138
Individualized Education Program (IEP), 78, 192
Industry
    communication disorders and, 38
    counseling and, 43–45
    versus inferiority (Erikson model), 35
Inferiority versus industry, 35, 38
Information and group process, 125–126
Information model of counseling, 1–4, 64–65

Initiative
 counseling and, 42–43
 versus guilt (Erikson model), 35
Initiative norm, 132
Institution-centered diagnosis, 77–79, 89–91
Integration stage of coping process, 71–72
Integrity
 counseling and, 48–49
 versus despair (Erikson model), 37
Interaction norm, 131–132
Interpersonal learning
 and groups, 126–127
 and training of clinicians, 183–189
Intimacy
 counseling and, 47
 in families, 175
 versus isolation (Erikson model), 36–37
Isolation versus intimacy, 36–37
Israelite, N. K., 171
Itzkowitz, J., 109
Jackson, Don, 146
Jargon, 3, 63–64
Jewell, Geri, 24
Johns, J., 108
Johnson, P., 147–148
Johnson, W., 187
Joy
 of parents, 66
 of professionals, 66–67
Kabat-Zinn, J., xviii
Kasprisin-Burrell, S., 147–148
Kazak, A., 162
Keane, K., 161
Keane-Hagerty, E., 23
Keller, Helen, 56–57
Keller, Mrs., 56–57, 194
Keogh, B., 176
Kierkegaard, Søren, 18
Kinsley, Emily Perle, 54–55
Klevans, D., 184–185
Kommers, M. S., 150
Kopp, Sheldon, 15, 40
Kornhaber, C., 167
Krueger, S., 2, 78
Kubler-Ross, E., 53, 98
Kupferer, S., 23
Kurtzer-White, E., 90

Land, S. L., 109
Language Changing technique, 110–111

Lao-tze, 15
Larson, M., 3
Laryngectomees, 3, 25, 132, 150
Lash, J. V., 56–57
Lavell, N., 176
Leadership
 confrontation and, 133–134, 137–138
 functions of, 130–131
 in groups, 130–135
 here–and–now norm and, 134
 initiative norm and, 132
 interaction norm and, 131–132
 procedural norms and, 135
 respect for individual needs and, 134–135
 self-disclosure and, 132–133
Lear, M., 46
Lecture (teaching device), 43–44
Leichook, A., 148–149, 192
Lerner, W., 2–3, 79
Letting go, 180
Leventhal, J., 97
Lieberman, M., 130, 140
Life cycle model (Erikson)
 communication disorders and, 38–39
 existentialism and, 49
 relationship building and, 39–49
 stages of, 33–37
Lloyd, L., 14
Lobato, D., 171
Locus of control, 108–110, 187
Loneliness, 21–22, 25–26
Love, 22
Love's Executioner (Yalom), 19
Lowe, T., 167
Lucks, L., 2, 181–182
Lund, N. J., 148
Luterman, David M., xv, 90, 141, 172

Madison, L., 109
Malone, R. L., 149–150
Manolson, A., 149
Marriage, 151–154. See also Divorce; Families;
 Parents
Martin, E., 2, 78, 79
Marvin, R., 162
Maslow, Abraham, 15
Massie, Bobby, 25–26
Massie, Suzanne, 25–26
Matis, E., 148
Matkin, N., 157

Matson, D., 67
Mattingly, M. A., 190
Maxwell, D., 29
May, R., 6, 195
May, Rollo, 18
McCarthy, P., 2, 181-182
McKee, B., 108
McKelvey, J., 124
Meadow, K., 38–39, 189–190
Meaninglessness, 22–23, 26–27
Medical model
  of counseling, 1–6
  of diagnosis, 77–78
Medoff, Mark, 187
Mendel, L., 2, 182
Mendelsohn, M., 155
Mental retardation, 79–80
Metz, D., 124
Miles, M., 130
Miller, M., 183
Minnesota Multiphasic Personality Inventory
  (MMPI), 182–183
Minuchin, Salvador, 146, 147, 154, 169
The Miracle Worker, 56–57, 58
Mistakes in counseling, 51–52, 86, 115, 118–122
Mistrust versus trust, 34, 38, 39–41
Mitford, J., 19
MMPI (Minnesota Multiphasic Personality Inventory), 182–183
Models as clinical tools, 49. See also Life cycle
  model (Erikson)
Modification strategy for coping, 73
Moliere, 23
Montague, J., 13–14
Morrison, E., 17, 184
Mosak, H., 24
Moustakes, C., 22, 26
Multiculturalism, 193
Munro, J., 24
Murphy, Albert, 17, 189
The Nature of Suffering and the Goals of Medicine
  (Cassell), xviii
Needham, C., 161
Negative reinforcement, 12
Novak, C., 178
Nuland, S. D., 124, 165–166

O'Connor, S., 124
Olson, D., 174
Olswang, L. B., 193

Operant conditioning, 12–14
Optimal families
  characteristics of, 174–176
  research on successful families, 176–180
Over–helping, 24–25, 57–58, 121, 183, 194

Palmer, C., 167
Parents. See also Families
  anger of, 58–61, 157–158
  children of parents with disability, 162–166
  denial by, 67–70, 80, 82, 86
  emotions of, 8–9, 157–159
  grief of, 48, 52–55, 83, 84, 158–159
  guilt of, 62, 158, 168
  IEP and, 192
  inadequacy feelings of, 55–58
  involvement of, in diagnosis, 80–88
  joy of, 66
  professional–parent relationships, 188–189
  resistance by, 70–71
  role of, 45–46, 154–162
  self–esteem of, 177–178
  vulnerability of, 62–63
Pavlov, Ivan, 11–12
Pearlin, L., 72
Peck, Scott, 22
Pedersen, F., 155
Perkins, W.P., 13
Personal growth
  and group process, 129
  and training of clinicians, 183–189
Persuasion model of counseling, 4–6, 31
Pickering, M., 184
Positive reinforcement, 12
Post, Joysa, 40
Potter, R., 183
Priddy, M., 124
Primus, M., 2
Procedural norms of groups, 135
Projection, 119–120
Psychosomatic illnesses, 147
Public schools, counseling in, 3–4, 191–192
Punishment, 12
Rabins, P., 165
Rational-emotive therapy, 28–29
Reflective silence, 113
Reframing
  as coping strategy, 74
  as counseling technique, 98–99
Reid, M., 14

Reinforcement, 12
Rescue syndrome, 24–25, 57–58, 121, 183, 194
Resistance
  as coping stage, 70–71
  group process and, 138
Respect for individual needs, 134–135
Responsibility/freedom, 20–21, 24–25
Rigrodsky, S., 17, 184
Rimm, D. C., 12
The Road Less Traveled (Peck), 22
Robertson, E., 148
Rogers, Carl, 15–16, 97, 142, 184, 195
Role confusion versus identity, 35–36, 38–39
Rollins, W., 87, 153–154
Romantic love, 22
Roosevelt, Eleanor, xvi
Rosman, B., 147
Rotter, S., 108
Rotter Locus of Control scale, 108, 187
Roy, R., 164
Rozek, E., 155
Ruscello, D., 188
Russell, Bertrand, 66
Russell, C., 174

Sabbeth, B., 97
Sager, C., 151
Salloway, S., 23
Sandow, S., 177
Satir, Virginia, 146–147, 155
Scharfman, W., 155
Schein, J., 124
Schlessinger, H., 38–39, 177
Schmitt, M., xvi, 3–4
Schooler, S., 72
Schools. See Public schools
Schwirian, P., 171
Science and Human Behavior (Skinner), 12
Self-actualization, 15
Self-disclosure, 132–133
Self-esteem of parents, 177–178
Seligman, M., 124, 171
Setting of group, 142
Shame versus autonomy, 34–35, 38, 41–42
Shames, G., 13, 147–148
Sharing self, 99–100
SHHH (Self Help for Hard of Hearing People), 71
Shirlberg, L., 109
Shlien, J., 24
Siblings, 169–174. See also Families

Silence, 111–113
Singler, J., 124
Size of group, 142
Skinner, B. F., 12
Smith, J., 124
Spanish–American War veterans, 69–70
Special Children, Special Parents (Murphy), 189
Speech–language pathologists. See also Counseling
  certification of, 188
  counseling skills of, 3–4
  diagnosis by, 87
  emotions of, 65–67
  group process used by, 123–124
  and limits of counseling, 193–195
  multiculturalism and, 193
  parent programs and, 188–189
  training and education for, 2, 181–189
Spina bifida, 162
Spouses, 58–61, 151–154. See also Families
Spradlin, J., 14
Sprenkle, D., 174
Stagnation versus generativity, 37
Starkweather, C., 14
Stavis, R., 32
Stech, E., 14
Stereotyping, 119
Stevenson, Robert Louis, 21
Stone, J., 193, 194
Stress in families, 179–180. See also Coping process
Stress reduction, 74–75. See also Coping process
Stroke patients, 27, 148
Structured experiences and groups, 140–141
Stutterers
  behavior modification of, 13
  cognitive therapy for, 29
  counseling for, 7
  family therapy with, 147–148
  humanistic counseling for, 17
  locus of control and, 109
  loneliness of, 25
Sudden inception diagnosis, 89–91
Suinn, R., 148
Sullivan, Annie, 56–57, 194
Sullivan, M. D., 150
Superior, K., 148–149, 192
Sweetow, R., 5

Tanner, D. C., 53
Tarver, S., 109

Tattersall, H., 83
Termination
    of group, 139–140
    integrity and, 48
Termination silence, 113
Therapists. *See* Counseling
Throne, S., 13–14
Thurman, Robert, xix
Tinkleberg, J., 124
Training in counseling
    for clinical competence and personal growth,
        183–189
    for clinicians, 2, 181–183
    for humanistic counseling, 184
    importance of, 181–182
    locus of control and, 109
    parent–professional relationships and, 188–
        189
Transactional analysis, 24–25
Transference, 119
Trivette, C., 174
Troesch, P., 14
Trust
    communication disorders and, 38
    in counseling, 39–41, 97
    versus mistrust (Erikson model), 34

Universality, 125

Van Kleeck, A., 193
Van Riper, C., 184, 185
Vance, B., 27
Venters, M., 176

Ventimiglia, R., 152–153
Veterans Administration, 69–70
Vineberg, S. E., 109
Voeller, M., 174
Volz, H., 184–185
Vulnerability
    of clients, 62–63
    of professionals, 66

Ward, B., 183–184
Warner, R., 32
Watson, John, 11
Webster, E., 8, 17, 124, 183–184
Webster, M., 24, 149
Wexler, K., 124
Wherever You Go, There You Are (Kabat–Zinn),
    xviii
Whitaker, Carl, 146
White, K., 24, 108
White, S., 1
Wiggins, E., 186
Wilkin, C., 23
Williams, D. M. L., 2, 79
Woodward, L., 167
Working group stage, 138–139
Wright, David, 20

Yalom, I., 18, 19–20, 23, 32, 125, 128, 130, 135,
    140, 159
Yarnell, G., 14
Young, A., 83

Zeine, L., 3

ABOUT THE AUTHOR

David M. Luterman, EdD, is professor emeritus at Emerson College in Boston and director of the Thayer Lindsey Family Centered Nursery for Hearing Impaired Children. He has dedicated his career to developing a greater understanding of the psychological effects and emotions associated with hearing impairment and the caregiver role. He has successfully translated this understanding into a model of counseling that allows for content and affect exchange. He has written and lectured extensively on counseling throughout the United States, Canada, and abroad. He is a fellow of the American Speech-Language-Hearing Association. He is author of *Counseling Parents of Hearing Impaired Children* (1979, Little, Brown), *Deafness in Perspective* (1986, College Hill), *Deafness in the Family* (1987, College Hill), *In the Shadows* (1995, Jade Press), *The Young Deaf Child* (1999, York Press), *Early Childhood Deafness* (co-edited with Ellen Kurtzer-White, York Press, 2001), *When Your Child Is Deaf* (2001, York Press), and *Hearing Loss in Children: A Family Guide* (Auricle Ink Press, 2006).